Obstetric Anaesthesia: Anaesthesia in a Nutshell

Commissioning editor: Melanie Tait
Development editor: Zoë A. Youd
Production controller: Chris Jarvis
Desk editor: Claire Hutchins
Cover designer: Alan Studholme

Obstetric Anaesthesia: Anaesthesia in a Nutshell

David Vaughan MBBS FRCA
Consultant Anaesthetist, Northwick Park and St Mark's Hospital, Watford Road, Harrow, Middlesex, UK

Neville Robinson MBChB FRCA
Consultant Anaesthetist, Northwick Park and St Mark's Hospital, Watford Road, Harrow, Middlesex, UK

Series Editors: **Neville Robinson and George Hall**

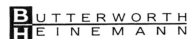

OXFORD AUCKLAND BOSTON JOHANNESBURG MELBOURNE NEW DELHI

Butterworth-Heinemann
Linacre House, Jordan Hill, Oxford OX2 8DP
225 Wildwood Avenue, Woburn, MA 01801-2041
A division of Reed Educational and Professional Publishing Ltd

ℛ A member of the Reed Elsevier plc group

First published 2002

© Reed Educational and Professional Publishing Ltd 2002

British Library Cataloguing in Publication Data
A catalogue record for this book is available from the British Library

Library of Congress Cataloguing in Publication Data
A catalogue record for this book is available from the Library of Congress

ISBN 0 7506 5008 7

For information on all Butterworth-Heinemann
publications visit our website at www.bh.com

Transferred to digital printing in 2006.

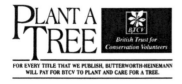

Contents

Series preface

Specialist registrars and senior house officers in anaesthesia are now trained by the use of modular educational programmes. In these short periods of intense training the anaesthetist must acquire a fundamental understanding of each anaesthetic specialty. To meet these needs, the trainee requires a concise, pocket-sized book that contains the core knowledge of each subject.

The aims of these 'nutshell' guides are two-fold: first, to provide trainees with the fundamental information necessary for the understanding and safe practice of anaesthesia in each specialty; and secondly, to cover all the key areas of the fellowship examination of the Royal College of Anaesthetists and so act as revision guides for trainees.

P. N. Robinson
G. M. Hall

Preface

One of the biggest challenges for the trainee anaesthetist is the transition from senior house officer to specialist registrar. Obstetric anaesthesia becomes a special hurdle in that the trainee, often with limited experience in the field, has to undertake extra responsibility. In obstetrics, this often occurs in an isolated environment.

Obstetric anaesthetic textbooks are invariably large and expensive. Our trainees have continuously stressed the need for a cheap, pocket-sized book that acts as a short, practical guide for safe anaesthetic practice in the delivery suite. They also wish for a book that will act as a basic source of reference to assist them in passing the Fellowship of the Royal College of Anaesthetists.

The drug dosages suggested help us practise this specialty safely, but are only a guide for the trainee. We realise that individual obstetric anaesthetic units have their own guidelines and drug regimens.

The topics follow the recommendations of training requirements made by the Obstetric Anaesthetists' Association and the Royal College of Anaesthetists. We have produced this text with these aims in mind, and hope that it achieves these ideals.

We wish to thank Drs Adrian Wagstaff, Anna Wilson and Joe Sebastian for their suggestions, and for assisting with the clear presentation of the text.

David Vaughan
Neville Robinson

List of boxes

Applied obstetric physiology

Pregnancy is an adaptive multisystem maternal response that allows fetal growth to occur in the best possible environment. The physiology of pregnancy is becoming understood in increasingly clear detail, and this chapter provides a brief overview of this process.

Cardiovascular

The increase in cardiac work in pregnancy is due primarily to the increased tissue oxygen requirements of both the mother and the fetus (Box 1.1).

The initial rapid rise in cardiac output does not continue throughout pregnancy. The increased pre-load and fall in after-load may produce functional heart murmurs – a systolic ejection murmur is common, and third and fourth heart sounds are

---

Box 1.1. Cardiovascular changes in pregnancy

- Maternal cardiac output rise is detectable at 6 weeks' gestation, and output has risen by 20 per cent at 10 weeks. At 34 weeks' gestation, maternal cardiac output is increased by 30–40 per cent. There is no change after this. The initial rise is primarily due to an increased heart rate (10–15 beats per minute). At term the rise is sustained by increases in both heart rate and stroke volume (cardiac muscle hypertrophy). In labour, output increases by an extra 30 per cent at the peak of maternal pushing.
- Central venous and pulmonary capillary wedge pressures are unchanged in a normal pregnancy.
- Systolic blood pressure is largely unchanged, but as the vascular resistance falls there is an accompanying fall in maternal diastolic blood pressure (evident in second trimester).
- The heart increases in size and is displaced left and anteriorly. The apex beat is displaced superolaterally due to upwards displacement of the diaphragm.
- Aortocaval compression occurs in the third trimester.

occasionally heard. There may be a bruit down the edge of the sternum over the course of the hypertrophied internal mammary artery. The cardiac outline is altered on a normal chest radiograph. The ECG shows ventricular hypertrophy (left > right), and the unfolding of the heart on the aortic and pulmonary tracts results in inverted T waves in V_2 and occasionally V_3. This is shown as an apparent left axis deviation.

Aortocaval compression

Aortocaval compression occurs to some degree in all women in the third trimester when in the supine position. The uterus obstructs the inferior vena cava, and there can be as much as a 22 per cent fall in cardiac output. The mother may not voluntarily reveal this. An alternative venous pathway via the paravertebral and azygos veins exists, which explains why women do not all present with the supine hypotensive syndrome of pregnancy. Many mothers will not lie in the supine position unless requested by medical staff to do so. The diminished venous return in this position may compromise cardiac output to the mother and fetus. The mother may be asymptomatic, but light-headedness, vomiting, dizziness and even unconsciousness can occur, as can fetal distress. The syndrome is worsened by contractions. It is wise to avoid the supine position for all term pregnant women and to place them in a left lateral position or tilted with a wedge.

Blood volume and coagulation

The blood volume increases in an almost linear fashion throughout pregnancy to a maximum at about 32 weeks. The increase in plasma volume (due to increased plasma water) is greater than the increase in red cell mass (40 per cent compared to 12 per cent at term). This relative haemodilution used to be called 'physiological anaemia'. The haemoglobin concentration drops from 13 g/dl in the non-pregnant state to about 11 g/dl at term. Most pregnant women in the UK are given iron and folate supplements. Iron requirements increase significantly due to greater maternal demand on top of huge fetal requirements. Folate is recommended (400 µg/day) for at least 3 months prior to conception and during the first trimester, to decrease the incidence of fetal neural tube defects. Box 1.2 lists the major haematological and biochemical changes.

The trend toward hypercoagulability is protective, decreasing the risk of haemorrhage at delivery. This is offset by the increased risk

---

Box 1.2. Blood volume and coagulation changes

- There is increased plasma volume and red cell mass but no compensatory plasma protein increase, resulting in a net decrease in packed cell volume and viscosity. ESR increases to 80 mm/h after delivery.
- Plasma cholinesterase concentration is reduced to 30 per cent of normal at term (this is of no clinical significance with suxamethonium or local anaesthetic esters).
- Electrolytes are unchanged.
- There is a trend towards a hypercoagulable state – platelet function and numbers are normal in health, there are increases in all coagulation factors (especially fibrinogen and VII), and plasminogen activation is slightly decreased. Bleeding, clotting and clot retraction times are all unchanged in health.

---

of deep vein thrombosis in pregnancy. At delivery there is increased fibrinolytic activity and high levels of plasminogen activators occur within the uterus, and these factors can cause disseminated intravascular coagulation.

Respiratory

In early pregnancy, progesterone causes women to breathe more deeply but not more frequently. Alveolar minute ventilation is doubled. Later, the expanding uterus increases the intra-abdominal pressure, causing the lower ribs to flare out. Expiratory reserve volume is decreased but minute volume is maintained as a result of an increase in rate. The changes are summarized in Box 1.3.

It is important to note that in the third trimester the closing volume may encroach upon the tidal volume in the supine position, in the very obese and in those with non-singleton pregnancies. Apnoea produces cyanosis more quickly in pregnancy for three reasons; oxygen consumption is increased, FRC is reduced, and airway closure may be present. This has important implications for general anaesthesia in that preoxygenation must be meticulous – even well oxygenated patients can desaturate during an uncomplicated intubation.

Gastrointestinal

There are two main gastrointestinal changes in pregnancy; smooth muscle relaxation from the effects of progesterone and relaxin, and the consequences of the expanding uterus. These result in prolonged

---

Box 1.3. Respiratory changes in pregnancy

Anatomical:

- There is diaphragmatic elevation of 4 cm.
- The anteroposterior and lateral diameters of the chest cavity are increased, and the chest circumference is increased by 5–7 cm.
- The substernal angle is increased.
- Diaphragmatic breathing.

Functional:

- At term, the functional residual capacity (FRC) is reduced by 20 per cent, the inspiratory reserve is increased by 20 per cent and the vital capacity is unchanged.
- The airway resistance decreases, lung compliance is unaffected, chest wall compliance reduces, and diffusion capacity is unchanged.
- Minute ventilation increases from 12 weeks, with a peak increase of 50 per cent at term. There is a rise in tidal volume and a small increase in rate. $PaCO_2$ is reduced by 20 per cent (4 kPa) and PaO_2 increased by 10–15 per cent.
- Oxygen consumption is increased by 20 per cent at term and over 100 per cent in the active second stage of labour.

---

gastrointestinal transit time and slower gastric emptying, and constipation is more common. Lower oesophageal sphincter tone is reduced, and reflux is common in the second and third trimesters. As the uterus expands, the stomach axis changes from vertical to horizontal and the intragastric pressure rises to twice that in the non-pregnant state. Up to 70 per cent of women complain of heartburn and all are at risk of regurgitation in labour. Opioids further delay gastric emptying, as do pain, anxiety and the supine position. The liver maintains normal size and blood flow. Albumin production is decreased, and with the increased plasma volume drug pharmacokinetics and dynamics may be altered.

Renal

The increased circulating volume causes a 40 per cent increase in renal blood flow and in the glomerular filtration rate. This is accompanied by enhanced tubular absorption; plasma concentrations of urea and creatinine decrease to 50 per cent and 66 per cent of the non-pregnant levels respectively. The maximal tubular resorption threshold for creatinine, glucose and uric acid is reduced. Intermittent glycosuria and orthostatic proteinurea can occur in normal pregnancies. Progesterone relaxes the muscle of the bladder. The muscle walls of the ureters become larger and wider, and are of lower tone. Ureteric stasis can occur, increasing the risk of urinary infection. Frequency of micturition is common, caused by mechanical compression of the bladder by the enlarging uterus.

Endocrine

All maternal endocrine function is altered in pregnancy, mainly as a result of the increased pituitary gland trophic hormone production (Box 1.4). The pituitary gland venous portal system is at full capacity at term. A drop in perfusion (classically due to a postpartum haemorrhage) may lead to pituitary infarction – Sheehan's syndrome.

Genital tract

The increased bulk of the uterus is due mainly to hypertrophy (20-fold) of the myometrial cells. This growth is stimulated by oestrogen. At term, the blood flow through the uterine and ovarian arteries is 1.0–1.5 l/min. The placenta is preferentially perfused, with 85 per cent of the flow directed to the uterus.

Epidural and spinal compartments

The epidural veins, which are thin walled and valveless, are distended in pregnancy. They form part of an important alternative

---

Box 1.4. Endocrine changes in pregnancy

Pituitary gland:
- Anterior – prolactin and adrenocorticotrophic hormone are increased, follicle stimulating hormone, luteinizing hormone and growth hormone are decreased, thyrotrophin is unchanged.
- Posterior – oxytocin via the hypothalamus increases in labour (lower genital tract stretching, and suckling).

Thyroid gland:
- The basal metabolic rate is increased.
- T_3 and T_4 are increased.
- The patient is clinically euthyroid.

Adrenal glands:
- Plasma cortisol and rennin are raised.
- Adrenaline and noradrenaline are unchanged, but rise in labour.

pathway for venous return in patients who are in the supine position. The volumes of both the epidural and subarachnoid spaces are reduced as a result of the increased size in the epidural veins. The epidural pressure is unchanged in pregnancy but increases during contractions. In active second stage pushing, this rises to 4–10 cmH$_2$O. The cerebrospinal fluid alters minimally in pregnancy – the specific gravity and total protein are slightly lower. The net result for regional analgesia is that in the last trimester, less local anaesthetic is required (about two-thirds of the non-pregnant dose). This effect is due to venous engorgement reducing the apparent volume of the epidural and intrathecal spaces. These effects decrease to normal levels after 3 days.

Weight gain

The average weight gain throughout pregnancy is about 12 kg, and the basal metabolic rate at term is increased by about 15 per cent.

2

Labour and the fetus

Labour is a process that, at its simplest, is entirely natural and requires no medical intervention. Increasingly high degrees of intervention by obstetric, paediatric and anaesthetic staff are now required to enable more complex pregnancies to come to fruition. A basic understanding of the process and management of normal labour and its effects on the fetus is crucial when dealing with abnormal labour.

Initiation of labour

The endocrine factors that initiate labour are still not fully understood. It is known that contractions are triggered by an increase in cervical prostaglandin secretion, and this is related to an increase in cyclo-oxygenase pathway product receptors and oestrogen receptors in the uterine cervix. Artificial induction of labour is based on this knowledge, and is most commonly performed by the repeated application of prostaglandin gel or pessaries to the cervix.

Labour is regarded as active or under way once rhythmic, regular contractions are established. These increase in amplitude, frequency and level of discomfort, and may be accompanied by a 'show' of blood and mucus released from its plugging position in the canal of the now dilating cervix.

Stages of labour

First stage of labour

This is the period from the establishment of true labour to full dilation of the cervix. It can be subdivided into two phases: the steady, regular contractions causing cervical dilation to 6–7 cm; and the more painful and increasingly frequent transitional phase contractions where cervical dilation is accompanied by descent and rotation of the presenting part. The first stage is of variable length in primiparous mothers (mean duration 12 hours, median 10 hours, modal 9 hours; but often up to or over 24 hours), but in multiparous patients may only last 2–4 hours. Contractions are initiated in uterine fundal pacemaker cells and spread throughout the uterus. These contractions apply pressure onto the cervix via the forewaters in the amniotic sac if the membranes have not ruptured. This causes further prostaglandin release, which softens or 'ripens' the cervix.

The time between contractions shortens through labour such that initially they may be every 15 minutes but by the second stage they often come every 2 minutes.

Second stage of labour

Once the cervix is fully dilated the presenting part descends onto the pelvic floor and into the upper vagina. Contractions slow but greatly increase in intensity, and are accompanied by the urge to push, a reflex triggered by this pelvic floor pressure. The mother is encouraged to perform a Valsalva with each breath during the contractions, and cries of 'Push into your bottom!' are common in delivery units. This direct pressure along the long axis of the fetus enables the dilation of the birth canal until the head and subsequently the body are delivered.

The second stage lasts up to 2 hours, although it may be considerably less. Failure to deliver after this time usually necessitates obstetric intervention.

Third stage of labour

There is usually a period of 15–30 minutes of uterine inaction prior to contractions restarting to expel the placenta. As the use of ergometrine and oxytocin have now become routine, this rest period is often not seen. The placenta and membranes must be carefully inspected to ensure complete delivery from the uterus.

Assessment of labour

The mainstay of normal labour control is the midwife. Ideally, there should be one-to-one midwifery care for all labouring women. As well as assisting the mother through the rigours of childbirth, the role of the midwife has expanded over the last two decades to include assessment of labour progression via non-clinical means, and acting as the main interface between the patient and the medical services.

Vaginal examinations are usually performed 4-hourly to assess cervical dilation and fetal position and orientation. This may be more frequent if worries about the progress of labour or fetal well being exist. These findings are documented graphically on a partogram to provide a clear visual record of progression. 'Active' management of labour (the process by which the partogram is used to assess the need for intervention such as artificial membrane rupture and augmentation of labour with oxytocin infusions) is a process now beginning to fall out of use, superseded by a return to a more 'naturalistic' approach. Simple examination of the liquor may also reveal the presence of meconium – the freshness of the staining and its intensity are indicative of the timing and severity of fetal distress.

Cardiotocography provides a wealth of data during labour. It is a dual trace showing fetal heart rate (either recorded trans-abdominally using Doppler or directly via a fetal scalp electrode) in relation to uterine pressure (usually recorded indirectly via an abdominal strain gauge, but sometimes directly with an intrauterine balloon). The main points in CTG interpretation are summarized in Box 2.1.

Fetal capillary blood can be taken transvaginally during labour from the presenting part. This provides a direct measure of fetal tissue pH and is often the factor on which the decision to proceed to Caesarean section is made, a pH of less than 7.25 being evidence of

---

Box 2.1. The cardiotocograph (CTG): basic interpretation

- Heart rate: the normal range at >36 weeks is 120–160 beats per minute. Tachycardia (moderate <180, severe >180 beats per minute for 5 minutes) indicates possible fetal hypoxia, and fetal arrhythmia should be considered if it is prolonged or unprovoked. The degree of bradycardia (mild >100, moderate 80–100, severe <80 beats per minute for 5 minutes) usually mirrors the severity of fetal acidosis. The significance is greater if other CTG changes are also present. Maternal hypotension should be excluded.
- Beat-to-beat rate variability: this should be greater than seven. This reflects intact autonomic function, and loss may reflect early fetal hypoxia. A sleeping (non-active) fetus and drug effects (from pethidine, maternal blockade) should be excluded.
- Response to contraction: there is usually nil response or a mild rate acceleration. Early decelerations (prior to the peak in contraction pressure) may indicate tension on or obstruction of the umbilical cord, or may just be due to pressure on the fetal head. Late decelerations (after the contraction peak) are the clearest marker of fetal distress, especially if accompanied by a decrease in beat-to-beat variability. In each case, the severity is linked to the degree and duration of deceleration (i.e. the area of the dip).

significant distress and a pH of less than 7.2 indicating the need for immediate delivery.

Abnormal presentation

The commonest malpresentation is breech. This is usually diagnosed in late pregnancy, when external cephalic version (manual fetal rotation by external pressure) should be offered. This is successful in 40 per cent of primiparous mothers and 60 per cent of multiparous women. About 50 per cent of attempted vaginal breech deliveries are successful. This is more likely with smaller babies, a large pelvic inlet and outlet, multiparous mothers and senior obstetric staff.

Transverse lie is an absolute indication for Caesarean section if it fails to correct once labour has started.

Multiple pregnancy

Multiple pregnancy is becoming more common with the increasing use of fertility drugs and in vitro fertilization. Approximate figures for incidence in the UK are: twins 1 : 80; triplets 1 : 2000; and quadruplets 1 : 80 000. These present no particular anaesthetic challenge, although it must be remembered that regional block insertion may be technically more difficult as the mother is less able to flex her spine. During vaginal delivery the risks are greatest immediately after delivery of the first baby, as the relatively capacious uterine cavity permits malpositioning of the subsequent fetus, and cord prolapse may occur. Multiple deliveries have increased risk of haemorrhage due to uterine atony.

Fetal circulatory changes at birth

The fetus is totally dependent on the placenta for nutrition and respiration. Until the first breath is taken and the lungs expand, they are small, collapsed structures receiving only 3–4 per cent of the cardiac output. Oxygenated blood from the placenta enters the fetus via the umbilical vein (approximate oxygen saturation 80 per cent). Most of the blood passes to the inferior vena cava via the ductus venosus, thus bypassing the liver. A sphincter in the ductus venosus controls the proportion entering the liver sinusoids and mixing with portal blood. This closes during uterine contractions to prevent sudden heart failure due to the massive increase in venous return from the compressed placenta.

The blood from the inferior vena cava (approximate oxygen

Box 2.2. Changes in the fetal circulation at birth

- Umbilical artery closure: closure is caused by smooth muscle spasm within a few minutes of birth, and is triggered by the change in oxygen tension. The complete obliteration of the lumen takes several months, after which the proximal portions of the arteries form the medial umbilical ligaments, whilst the distal portions persist as the superior vesical arteries.
- Closure of umbilical vein and ductus venosus: this occurs after arterial closure to allow return of fetal blood from the placenta. After obliteration, the umbilical vein forms the ligamentum teres hepatis in the lower border of the falciform ligament. The ductus venosus becomes the ligamentum venosum.
- Closure of the ductus arteriosus: this occurs almost immediately after the first breath, due to wall muscle spasm triggered by bradykinin release from the expanding lung. Anatomical obliteration and conversion to the ligamentum arteriosum takes up to 3 months, and in premature infants hypoxia may cause the ductus to reopen, leading to a potentially fatal return to a fetal circulation.
- Closure of the foramen ovale: mechanical closure occurs with lung expansion as the left atrial pressure rises and right-sided pressure falls. This closure is reversible in the neonatal period (crying produces a right-to-left shunt, causing transient cyanosis), but constant apposition leads to fusion by about 1 year of age. Twenty per cent of people never achieve perfect anatomical closure (probe patent foramen ovale).

---

saturation 75 per cent) is guided through the foramen ovale into the left atrium. A small proportion remains in the right atrium, mixes with deoxygenated blood from the superior vena cava territory, and passes to the pulmonary trunk (approximate oxygen saturation 50 per cent) via the right ventricle. As the pulmonary vascular resistance is very high, most flows via the ductus arteriosus into the descending aorta.

The relatively oxygen-rich mixture in the left atrium passes to the ventricle and is ejected into the aorta. The coronary and carotid arteries leave the aorta proximal to the ductus arteriosus, ensuring the heart and brain are supplied with well-oxygenated blood. The blood in the descending aorta distal to the ductus arteriosus (approximate oxygen saturation 55 per cent) supplies the abdominal organs and lower limbs. Blood is returned to the placenta via the two umbilical arteries arising from the common iliac vessels.

The changes in the fetal circulation at birth are summarized in Box 2.2.

3

Drugs, the placenta and the fetus

All drugs used in medicine have the potential to produce both beneficial and harmful effects. This is particularly so in pregnancy and labour, where these effects have to be considered in two patients rather than one. This chapter covers placental drug transfer mechanisms, and pays specific reference to those drugs commonly used in pregnancy and labour.

Placental drug transfer
Diffusion
Factors affecting transplacental drug diffusion are summarized in Box 3.1. Lipophilic molecules (up to a molecular weight of about 1000) simply diffuse across the placenta. Hydrophilic molecules cross much less readily; only those with a molecular or atomic weight of under 100 are able to diffuse passively to any significant degree. Simple non-polar compounds (respiratory gases, inhalational anaesthetics) and those that can exist in a non-polar or non-ionized state (weak acids – thiopentone, non-steroidal anti-inflammatory drugs; weak bases – local anaesthetics, opioids) can cross the barrier easily. Drugs that contain a quaternary amine

---

Box 3.1. Factors affecting placental drug diffusion

- Permeability – the relative ease with which a drug is able to cross the single layer of chorion separating maternal and fetal blood.
- The concentration gradient between the maternal and fetal plasma.
- The blood flow, both maternal and fetal, through the placenta.
- The degree of drug protein binding.
- The duration of exposure to the drug (i.e. a single dose/infusion/ repeated doses).
- Fetal acidosis, which increases the pH gradient across the placenta and thus increases the ionization of basic drugs (this is especially of relevance with opioids and local anaesthetics) in the fetal circulation, hence increasing transfer rate and total plasma concentration.

group (muscle relaxants) are fully ionized in solution, and thus placental transfer is very slow and usually clinically irrelevant. Similarly, the transfer of highly protein-bound drugs is negligible compared to free lipophilic compounds.

Active processes

Essential compounds such as amino acids, glucose, nucleic acids and water-soluble vitamins require specialized rapid transfer across the placenta. Most are actively transferred against the concentration gradient via mechanisms powered by Na^+/K^+ ATPase pumps. Immunoglobulins cross via pinocytosis in the microvilli of the chorion. Glucose is transferred by an energy-neutral system called facilitated diffusion, which allows more rapid transfer along the maternal–fetal concentration gradient.

Regional blockade and placental perfusion

Placental blood flow is determined by the maternal blood pressure and localized vascular tone. Several factors may affect these variables (see Box 3.2), but with current practice moving rapidly towards selective, controlled low-dose or mobile regional block, these problems are less commonly seen. Fluid preloading does not prevent hypotension after epidural block. Indeed, this may also have the effect of delaying labour due to acute dilution of circulating prostaglandins and hormones. Ephedrine is the treatment of choice (bolus doses of 3–6 mg as required), as it has a predominant β_1-adrenoceptor agonist (positive inotropic and chronotropic) effect with this dose range. Alpha-adrenoceptor agonists (methoxamine, metaraminol and phenylephrine) act to raise blood pressure via vasoconstriction, thus reducing placental flow, and should be avoided prior to delivery.

Regional blockade also has beneficial effects on placental perfusion. The decrease in sympathetic outflow and catecholamine release gained with good analgesia significantly increases intervillous blood flow via arteriolar vasodilation, and is protective against progressive fetal and maternal metabolic acidosis. Epidural analgesia is often specifically requested in high-risk parturients for this reason.

Drug effects on the fetus/neonate

A good rule of thumb is to avoid drug use wherever possible in the pregnant patient. The first trimester in particular is a high-risk time,

---

Box 3.2. Factors affecting placental blood flow during regional analgesia

- Maternal blood pressure is often reduced initially when the epidural or spinal local anaesthetic is given due to acute reduction in outflow from the sympathetic chain.
- Maternal cardiac output falls dramatically if aortocaval compression occurs. This is more common with a dense ('high-dose') block, as the mother is less able to move about and tends to remain in a supine position.
- Vasopressors cause a direct decrease in placental blood flow.

---

as this is the period when organogenesis occurs and the fetus is most susceptible to mutagenic effects.

Teratogenesis

Anaesthetic drugs have been shown to produce morphological teratogenic effects in rabbits and rodents only after prolonged exposure at subanaesthetic concentrations or multiple exposures at anaesthetic concentrations. These changes are thought to be due to fetomaternal physiological alterations rather than a direct effect. The only possible exception to this is nitrous oxide, but the extreme conditions needed to produce these changes in the laboratory indicate no problem for the pregnant woman. Behavioural teratogenesis in animals occurs at lower concentrations and exposure times. However, it is difficult to apply these data across species. Certainly epidemiological studies have shown no morphological teratogenic effect, but neurobehavioural function in children at high prenatal exposure risk has not been assessed fully in studies to date.

Drugs

- The *intravenous agents* commonly used in obstetric anaesthesia (thiopentone 3–5 mg/kg and etomidate 0.3 mg/kg) are clinically harmless to the neonate. There is reasonably good evidence that propofol, either as an induction bolus or a maintenance infusion, causes significant neurobehavioural depression in the neonate, and possibly some depression of Apgar scores. Ketamine has no depressant effect at a dose of 1 mg/kg, but causes neonatal respiratory and behavioural depression in over 25 per cent of deliveries at a more usual dose of 2 mg/kg. This, combined with the maternal risks of dissociation, hallucinations and delirium, make it unsuitable except in situations where placental flow is severely compromised, when the haemodynamic benefits may outweigh the risks.

- *Benzodiazepines* are less commonly used in pregnancy and labour than in the past. Chronic use in early pregnancy is associated with cleft lip or palate development. Diazepam rapidly crosses the placenta and the drug and its metabolites persist in the fetus for days, leading to low Apgar scores, decreased heart rate variability, hypoactivity, hypotonia, poor feeding, impaired metabolic responsiveness and elevation of bilirubin levels. Given the widespread acceptance of magnesium for treatment of eclamptic seizures as well as prophylaxis against them, the use of diazepam in labour is now becoming questionable. Midazolam accumulates to a lesser degree in the fetus, but again it has no role that cannot be adequately fulfilled by another class of drug, and so perhaps its usage should be avoided.

- *Inhalational anaesthetics* readily cross the placenta, with fetal plasma concentrations of between 50 and 90 per cent of that found in the mother after equilibration. This effect is one of the reasons that the time from induction to delivery in a Caesarean section under general anaesthesia should be as short as possible to avoid fetal anaesthesia. However, nitrous oxide, isoflurane and sevoflurane are all rapidly excreted from the lungs by the neonate, and any sedation produced is transient. The use of 50 per cent nitrous oxide with 0.6–0.8 MAC of one of these agents has been said to affect placental perfusion by causing maternal myocardial depression and vasodilation. This is offset partly by the increase in placental flow caused by reduction in catecholamine-mediated stress responses in the fetus, decreasing fetal acidosis.

- *Opioid* effects vary widely due to differences in lipophilicity, acidity and protein binding. Pethidine has a much lower oil/water partition coefficient than fentanyl, and is 40–60 per cent protein bound. This is rather deceptive, however, as its bond with α-1 acid glycoprotein (the principal plasma carrier protein for pethidine) is weak and does not impair diffusion. It diffuses rapidly across the placenta, and more so in the presence of fetal acidosis as it is a weak base. The fetal concentrations of pethidine and its rather more toxic metabolite norpethidine rise for up to 3 hours post maternal dose, and make a major contribution to reduction in Apgar scores. Fentanyl has a very mild fetal depressant effect not usually measurable in terms of Apgar score change, and the effects of alfentanil, morphine and diamorphine are negligible when used in usual clinical doses. At cardiac anaesthetic dosage (over 10 μg/kg fentanyl), loss of beat-to-beat variability and bradycardia are seen.

- *Muscle relaxants* all contain a quaternary amine group, and thus do not have significant placental transfer. The only exception to this rule is gallamine, a muscle relaxant not used clinically now but often seen in multiple-choice papers for this reason.
- *Local anaesthetics* are weak bases of intermediate to high lipid solubility. Fetal/maternal plasma concentration ratios are under 0.5, and thus if no evidence of maternal toxicity is seen the fetus is safe also.
- *Antimuscarinic drugs* all cross the placenta readily except for glycopyrrolate, the only quaternary amine. They have no known deleterious effects on the neonate.
- *Non-steroidal anti-inflammatory drugs* may cause pulmonary hypertension in the fetus, and can trigger premature closure of the ductus arteriosus with prolonged use in the third trimester. They extend labour and may delay its onset. They may cause transferred impairment of platelet function in the neonate.
- *Anti-emetic drugs* are used to treat hyperemesis gravidarum in pregnancy. Antihistamines (cyclizine, promethazine) are regarded as safe to use. Phenothiazines should be avoided, as should domperidone, metoclopramide and 5-HT$_3$ antagonists unless under specialist advice.
- *Antimicrobial agents* present a wide variety of potentially harmful effects in early pregnancy. Penicillins and cephalosporins are safe to use, but other antimicrobials should only be selected if need outweighs risk, and after microbiological consultation.
- *Antihypertensive drugs* are widely and increasingly used in pregnancy as detection and active management of pregnancy-related hypertension improves. The traditional mainstays of therapy are methyldopa, less lipophilic β-blockers (e.g. atenolol, labetalol, esmolol) and hydralazine. Beta-blockers should be used with care, as there are reports of fetal bradycardia and heart block. Drugs used for the long-term treatment of hypertension may need review if the patient becomes pregnant. Thiazides cause relative hypovolaemia and a fall in placental perfusion in the mother, and thrombocytopenia, jaundice, hyponatraemia, and an increased risk of hypertension in adulthood for the fetus. Lipophilic β-blockers such as propanolol cause neonatal

growth retardation, hypoglycaemia, bradycardia and respiratory depression. ACE inhibitors affect fetal and neonatal cardio-vascular control and renal function, and calcium channel blockers may inhibit the progress of labour.

- *Inotropes* should be used with extreme care in the gravid patient, as the risks of altering placental blood flow are great. Continuous cardiotocographic monitoring is mandatory and flow Doppler is also useful to assess the adequacy of the placental blood supply.
- *Alpha-adrenoceptor agonists* are absolutely contraindicated antenatally, as they cause a proven dose-related fall in placental perfusion, leading to profound fetal distress.
- *Anticoagulants* are used antenatally as thromboembolic prophylaxis in high-risk patients, and also as part of the treatment protocol for recurrent miscarriage. In addition, mothers may be on long-term anticoagulant therapy for intercurrent disease such as valvular heart disease. Heparin is a large polar molecule and thus crosses the placenta poorly. For this reason heparin and, more commonly now, low molecular weight heparins are the anticoagulants of choice in pregnancy. Warfarin and the other coumarins are highly (98 per cent) plasma protein bound, and thus are largely restricted from crossing the placenta. However, coumarins cause fetal chondrodysplasia and microcephaly if used in the first trimester, and are associated with a huge increase in the risk of massive antepartum haemorrhage in the third trimester.

4

Antenatal anaesthetic considerations

Patients present to the anaesthetist either antenatally or in labour. It is best practice to anticipate problems rather than be presented with an unanticipated difficulty in the middle of the night. For this reason, many units run antenatal assessment clinics to facilitate liaison for mothers with anaesthetic or multispecialty problems.

Antenatal clinics
Most departments run specialist consultant-led antenatal clinics for the assessment of high-risk patients. These clinics are also available to women who wish to discuss any problems or anxieties that they have regarding anaesthesia. They fall broadly into three groups; labour (in particular epidural analgesia), Caesarean section, and medical conditions affecting pregnancy.

Labour and epidural analgesia
How much or how little to say often depends on the patient – some wish for minimal information and some demand complete knowledge. Patients should be encouraged to attend relevant antenatal classes. Epidural analgesia is the most effective method of pain relief in labour, and of course the catheter can be used to provide analgesia for any ongoing procedures. It is initially effective in about 90 per cent of patients following the first dose. However, some patients require an alteration in the dose or catheter adjustment before effective analgesia occurs. The problems of epidural analgesia need to be discussed. It is reasonable to state that there are contraindications to it, and it is essential to state that there is a risk of post dural puncture headache associated with the procedure. The incidence of this within the maternity unit should be less than 1 per cent and ideally much lower. It is suggested that mothers are told that the headache can range from mild to severe, that it is postural, that they may have difficulty getting out of bed to look after their baby, and that they may have photophobia. The natural history of the headache is that it lasts for up to a week but can be

well managed and, if the mother asks, the management can be explained in detail. It is sufficient to state that it will 'slow' down the postnatal recovery period but can be well treated. In-depth discussion may be required.

Patients often worry about aggravating existing or developing new backache after an epidural. The facts are that new backache develops in about one in three mothers after pregnancy. There are many causes for backache after delivery – posture in pregnancy, a prolonged first stage, an obstructed or prolonged second stage, instrumental delivery and the postnatal reversal of the relaxin-mediated ligamentous laxity, and of course the mother must carry and care for the newborn child. There have been numerous studies that state that back pain has the same incidence whether or not the mother has had an epidural. Epidurals are easily blamed but are very, very rarely the cause of back pain. Occasionally the epidural puncture site can cause pain, and this is the only pain that the anaesthetist should take responsibility for. The degree of difficulty or the number of bone contacts made by the anaesthetist does not increase the incidence of backache. It is not uncommon for mothers to complain to anaesthetists of transient numbness in the distribution of the nerves supplying the legs. This is often in the distribution of the lateral cutaneous nerve of the thigh, and is almost always due to weight gain, the duration of labour and the mode of delivery. It is easy to blame the epidural, but it is rarely at fault. Although obstetricians usually assume anaesthetic responsibility, we are rarely the causal agents!

Patients worry about paralysis after an epidural. Rare isolated cases have occurred which have been proven to be due to misman-agement of the epidural, normally when neurolytic drugs are given in error. It is sufficient to state that correctly managed epidurals do not cause paralysis. It is generally agreed that there is an association between epidural analgesia and prolonged first and second stages of labour, forceps deliveries, and possibly Caesarean section. This does not mean that epidural analgesia causes the above – it is associated with those factors.

Some patients present saying they don't want an epidural. Choice is a mother's right, but it is worth asking why and also reassuring mothers that if they change their mind in labour they won't be refused one. Some patients present pre-labour to demand an epi-dural with the first contraction. It is sensible to tell them that it will be performed as soon as possible and that most units aim to provide epidural analgesia within 30 minutes of a maternal request. Ideally there is 24-hour cover devoted to the maternity unit, and this is what all units should aim for. Often there are two anaesthetists on site and more complete care can be given (even consultants can do labour epidurals!). Some mothers have had previous bad experiences of labour, unsympathetic midwives or anaesthetists, or bad epidural experiences, and need to be managed in an appropriate caring way.

Caesarean section

Assessment of patients for elective and emergency Caesarean section often falls to the trainee. Most (up to 90 per cent in many units) elective and emergency operations are carried out using regional anaesthesia, and the advantages of this are summarized in Box 4.1.

The advantages and disadvantages of general anaesthesia are summarized in Box 4.2.

Occasionally mothers will insist on general anaesthesia as their preference. This needs careful discussion, and their right to choice needs to be respected. If, however, general anaesthesia appears to be a dangerous and unsafe option, the risks must carefully be explained so that a sensible decision can then be made. An obstetric anaesthetist in an isolated unit often feels alone, and it is important

---

Box 4.1. Advantages and disadvantages of regional anaesthesia for Caesarean section

Advantages:
- Avoidance of complications of general anaesthesia.
- Better maternal experience of birth.
- Birthing partner present.
- Minimal drug transfer to fetus.
- Earlier mobilization.
- Less risk of chest infection.
- Less incidence of deep vein thrombosis.
- Better provision of postoperative analgesia.

Disadvantages:
- May be slower to set up.
- Surgeon preference for general anaesthesia in complicated cases.
- Patient preference for general anaesthesia.
- Complications of technique (hypotension, headache).
- Failure of regional technique (not effective, missed segment).

Box 4.2. Advantages and disadvantages of general anaesthesia for Caesarean section

Advantages:

- May be faster.
- Patient preference.
- Surgical preference.
- Airway controlled.
- No regional anaesthesia complications.

Disadvantages:

- Potential awareness.
- Potential hypoxia.
- Risk of intubation failure.
- Hypertensive response to intubation.
- Uterine relaxation.
- Drug transfer to fetus – lower Apgar scores due to sedation.
- More nausea and vomiting.
- More postoperative pain with slower recovery.
- Slower mobilization.
- Increased risk of chest infection.

---

to remember that assistance is always available. Often a mother's main concern is the fact that she will not be able to cope with the stress of being awake, and the thought of 'a needle in her back' often worries her most of all. These fears can normally be easily allayed.

Medical disease

Medical disease can either coexist with or be caused by pregnancy and its complications. Diabetes is an example of both. Management is normally via an insulin sliding-scale pump. Gestational diabetics usually revert to a non-diabetic state immediately following birth. Patients with chronic neurological disease such as multiple sclerosis can have regional anaesthesia, although some patients tend to blame any exacerbation of their disease on the epidural. This is unfounded. Cardiac conditions are high risk and should be managed with senior and cardiological advice. Peripartum cardiomyopathy can be serious and intensive care advice must be sought. Patients with respiratory disease should be treated with regional techniques by choice. In the United Kingdom, patients with cardiac, neurological and respiratory disease should be reported to the Obstetric Anaesthetist's Association Registry.

Consent

Problems often arise over complaints regarding the failure to provide prompt epidural analgesia, post dural puncture headache, and pain during Caesarean section. The patient must receive relevant information, have the opportunity to express her views, and know that her wishes will be respected. Complications with a greater than 1 per cent risk must be explained. In labour, patients with pain and those who have received drugs may or may not be able to give informed consent. Some units have written consent forms whilst others have verbal consent only. There is no right or wrong approach medicolegally. Consent simply is: 'if after explanation of the main indications and complications of a procedure the client cooperates, allowing the procedure to occur, then consent is seen to have been given'.

5

Analgesia for labour I: regional analgesia

Regional analgesia is without doubt the most effective form of pain relief for the labouring woman. This is provided in two main ways; by epidural administration of local anaesthetics, or by spinal (subarachnoid) injection of local anaesthetic with subsequent epidural top-ups if required. This analgesic benefit comes at a potentially high price: these techniques may result in serious and possibly fatal complications. Thus, the presence of a suitably trained anaesthetist with full resuscitation equipment to hand is mandatory in any delivery suite offering a regional analgesic service. However, the use of epidurals and combined spinal-epidurals (CSE) has revolutionized labour and delivery, and greatly facilitated obstetric interventions such as assisted delivery and Caesarean section.

Maternal pain transmission during childbirth
The pain felt during labour and delivery arises via two separate afferent pathways. The pain of uterine contractions and cervical dilation is carried via visceral afferent fibres through the uterine, cervical and hypogastric plexi to the sympathetic chain, and then via the white rami communicantes to the posterior nerve roots of T_{11}, T_{12} and L_1. During the progression through the transitional phase into the second stage of labour, the descent of the presenting part into the vagina and the associated stretching of the birth canal generates a second locus of pain. This is transmitted by the pudendal nerves and the perineal branches of the posterior cutaneous nerve of the thigh to the S_2, S_3 and S_4 nerve roots. In addition, somatic fibres from the cutaneous branches of the ilioinguinal and genitofemoral nerves carry afferent fibres to L_1 and, to a variable degree, L_2. Thus a spinal or epidural placed in the middle to lower lumbar region is ideal to cover both these nerve root groups, and can provide analgesia throughout labour and delivery.

Epidural analgesia

As previously stated, a block extending from T_{11} to S_4 is required for effective pain relief throughout labour. When an epidural is requested, it is the responsibility of the anaesthetist to ensure that the procedure is appropriate and safe, and that the patient understands the process and the more common potential problems. The indications and contraindications are summarized in Boxes 5.1 and 5.2.

Epidural insertion

When a patient requests an epidural, the anaesthetist has several considerations prior to performing the procedure. The medical and obstetric history must be ascertained relevant to any potential contraindications. Informed oral consent is vital. Procedural consent is assumed if the mother willingly permits the process to occur, but 'informed' consent is more difficult to quantify. The authors' practice is to warn of the risk of headache, discomfort, low blood pressure and partial or complete failure of the block. It is also stated that other complications exist which are rarer but potentially very serious, and that these can be further explained if the mother

---

Box 5.1. Epidural in labour: indications

- Pain – especially in prolonged labour and when incoordinate uterine contraction has been diagnosed. It should be considered based on pain severity, not cervical dilation.
- Breech presentation – it has been clearly shown that perinatal mortality decreases and Apgar scores and fetal pH are improved if an epidural is used in vaginal breech delivery.
- Multiple pregnancy – all complications of pregnancy are commoner in multiple births, with the greater risk being carried by the second twin. Epidural analgesia improves the acid–base state of the second twin and also facilitates operative delivery if necessary.
- Maternal cardiorespiratory and cerebrovascular disease – the avoidance of cardiorespiratory stress and opioids in those with significant cardiac or respiratory dysfunction will usually enable an assisted vaginal delivery to occur. The avoidance of straining and pushing with a planned instrumental delivery in those with cerebrovascular disease (such as aneurysmal vessels or arteriovenous malformations) decreases the risk of intracranial haemorrhage.
- Pre-eclampsia – complete analgesia stops the rise in mean arterial pressure, and may improve renal and placental blood flow.

Box 5.2. Epidural in labour: contraindications

Absolute:
- Allergy to local anaesthetic or analgesic drugs.
- Maternal refusal.
- Inability to establish large-bore intravenous access.
- Lack of resuscitation equipment or suitably trained staff.
- Coagulopathy.
- Septicaemia (as evidenced by temperature over 38°C, grossly raised/ abnormally low white cell count or evidence of infection-mediated organ dysfunction), or local infection at the site of insertion.

Relative – in all these cases epidurals can be sited, but it is recommended that trainee anaesthetists discuss with a senior colleague first:
- Relapsing neurological conditions (e.g. multiple sclerosis).
- Actively bleeding patients – cardiovascular stability must be established first.
- Fetal distress.
- Severe spinal deformity.

---

requests it. The mother is given a clear opportunity to ask questions. This is documented in the notes together with the procedure itself, and dosing and observational instructions. A large-bore intravenous cannula must be sited prior to injection of epidural drugs.

An increasingly common problem facing the obstetric anaesthetist is the patient who is a relative contraindication for epidural. Individual cases must be taken on their own merits, but if any doubt exists, the advice of a more senior colleague should be sought. A selection of these problem cases is outlined in Box 5.3, with management guidelines.

The following is an overview of epidural insertion; not a step-by-step guide to the uninitiated. The only way to learn how to site an epidural is to be taught by an expert senior colleague, and then to be assisted and supervised during progression up the learning curve.

The mother should be positioned in a way best suited to both parties – sitting or lying on the left side is equally acceptable. Strict aseptic technique should be used at all times. Gown and gloves are mandatory, and some units state that a hat and mask should also be worn. After the back has been prepped and draped, the spine is palpated to find the best space below Tuffiers' line (the imaginary line between the two iliac crests). Local anaesthetic (usually

---

Box 5.3. Grey areas for epidurals

Anticoagulants:

- Low-dose aspirin – not a problem; can be assessed if necessary with a formal bleeding time, but this is worthless unless performed properly by a trained observer.
- Unfractionated or low molecular weight heparins at prophylaxis dose – epidural should not be sited within 12 hours of the dose, although this may be reviewed if clinical need demands. Catheter removal should ideally be at least 6 hours before and after a dose.
- Fully anticoagulated (heparin/warfarin) – no.

Infection:

- Prolonged rupture of membranes – if apyrexial, normal white cell count and with clear liquor, yes. If any of the above are abnormal, discuss with a senior based on clinical indication.
- Localized, non-related infection (e.g. cold, chest infection) – yes.
- Systemic infection or sepsis – no.

Pre-eclampsia:

- Asymptomatic: platelet count 100 within the last 12–24 hours – yes. Platelet count 80–100 or falling over last few days – check clotting; if prothrombin time is normal – yes. Platelet count 80 – no.
- Symptomatic: check platelets and clotting as part of full blood screen. Discuss with senior based on results.

---

lignocaine 1–2%, 5 ml) is infiltrated into the skin and subcutaneous tissue. The Tuohy needle is then advanced into the epidural space, using a 'loss of resistance' technique. The catheter is then passed via the needle into the space, and positioned so that 3–5 cm is in the space when the needle has been removed. The catheter is aspirated to check for blood or CSF, and is then secured to the skin with sterile dressings.

Fluid preloading with 500–1000 ml Hartmann's solution or saline was mandatory in the recent past, but hypotension on induction of block is much less of a problem with low-dose epidural regimens. Evidence is quite clear that fluid bolus loading doesn't decrease the risk of hypotension, but may slow the rate and force of contractions (presumed to be due to an acute dilutional drop in maternal plasma levels of prostaglandins). However, local policy should be ascertained on arriving in a new delivery suite, and followed.

The air versus saline debate for loss of resistance has continued for many years, and is likely to do so for many more. Those who strongly promote air say that there is no chance of missing a dural tap if no fluid is injected into the epidural space and needle track during insertion. The only fluids seen at the needle hub with air are either blood or CSF, making diagnosis of vascular or dural puncture clear, and the only injectate used is local anaesthetic, decreasing the risk of inadvertent drug administration. Those in favour of saline argue that the continuous pressure technique used with it reduces the overall dural puncture rate, and that if the dura is breached 3–5 ml saline is not confused with a rush of warm CSF down a 16G needle. If doubt exists, assessment of the fluid with a glucose stick test gives a quick and reliable answer. Furthermore, they state that injecting air into the extradural space increases the risk of a patchy block (a bubble may form round a nerve root, preventing local anaesthetic contact and thus transmission blockade) and represents a small but significant infection risk. More obstetric anaesthetists use saline than air in UK practice today, but most accept that the skill of the operator is a far more important factor than the contents of the syringe, and both methods are acceptable.

Caudal analgesia is now rarely used in labour. Caudal single-shot or infusion techniques are clearly described in the historical literature. Technical difficulties, inadequacy of the block and infection risk mean that lumbar routes of access now supersede this.

Initiation of epidural analgesia

The amide local anaesthetic bupivacaine is by far the commonest epidural drug used in UK anaesthesia. With high-dose epidurals, it is standard practice to give a test dose to ensure positioning of an epidural catheter was correct prior to full block initiation, and 4 ml 0.5% bupivacaine ±1 : 200 000 epinephrine (1 ml in the filter and catheter; 3 ml in the epidural space; dose = 15 mg bupivacaine ±15 μg epinephrine) is often suggested. This will provide a full motor block without respiratory compromise if the catheter is placed intrathecally, and a rise in heart rate without cardiac compromise if it is in an epidural vein. This is then followed after 5–10 minutes by the analgesic dose of 5–10 ml bupivacaine 0.25%.

The introduction of low-dose epidurals has led to the concept of the first dose as both the analgesic and test dose. If the premise is accepted that a positive test dose indicates malplacement of the catheter but a negative test doesn't exclude it, then, provided suitable care and observation is taken throughout labour, this regimen is acceptable.

The low-dose or mobile epidural came about as a consequence of old-style epidurals leaving the mother pain free, but unable to move, feel her contractions or push effectively in the second stage. This in turn led to a midwifery practice of epidurals being left to wear off in the second stage to facilitate pushing. By using a much lower concentration of local anaesthetic in combination with a small dose of a lipophilic (to decrease systemic absorption) opioid such as fentanyl, a sensory blockade can reliably be established without motor loss. The incidence of hypotension also falls dramatically, and patchy blocks are less commonly a problem due to a more global spinal opioid effect.

The initial dose used to start a low-dose epidural varies from unit to unit. A selection of regimens used by the authors that fall into the 'tried and tested' category is shown in Box 5.4. The maintenance dose depends on technique and local policy. Most units use midwife-delivered bolus top-ups, but increasingly infusions with or without patient-controlled top-ups are being used. Box 5.5 describes the major fetomaternal effects of regional analgesia.

After initiation of block, 5-minute pulse and blood pressure checks should be carried out for at least 20 minutes. Cardiotocograph monitoring should also be applied, and care taken to ensure that aortocaval compression does not occur. Mothers may wish to walk about after epidural initiation. This is acceptable provided normal motor function is intact and the mother has a companion with her at all times.

Getting a block to work

Over 80 per cent of low-dose epidurals work effectively throughout labour with no problems. For those that do not produce adequate analgesia, solutions are usually easily found (see Box 5.6). It is vital when problems exist in initiating a block to accept early that the catheter is misplaced and to re-site the epidural rather than persist with larger volumes or higher concentrations of local anaesthetic. Thus it is important to check 15–20 minutes after the starter dose to assess if any analgesic effect is present. It is often the case that the block is merely at an inadequate height, and a further top-up dose is all that is needed to extend it and produce analgesia.

Where midwife-controlled top-ups are used it must be stressed to the mother that she should ask for an additional dose as soon as

---

Box 5.4. Suggested low-dose epidural starter and maintenance doses

---

Starting dose

- Bupivacaine 0.125% 10 ml + fentanyl 5 μg/ml (5 ml bupivacaine 0.25% + 1 ml neat fentanyl (50 μg) + 4 ml normal saline).
- Bupivacaine 0.1% 15 ml + fentanyl 2 μg/ml (3 ml bupivacaine 0.5% OR 6 ml bupivacaine 0.25% + 0.6 ml neat fentanyl (30 μg) + saline to 15 ml total; this dose is often available in premixed bags or syringes in the delivery suite).
- Ropivacaine 0.2% 10–15 ml.

Maintenance bolus dose

- Bupivacaine 0.1% + fentanyl 2 μg/ml, 10–15 ml of the mixture when needed (maximally every 20 minutes).
- Ropivacaine 0.2% 10 ml when needed (maximally every 20 minutes).

Maintenance infusion

- 10–20 ml/h of bupivacaine 0.1% + fentanyl 2 μg/ml OR ropivacaine 0.2%. Adjust infusion rate according to pain and block height; aim for between T_{10} (umbilicus) and T_6 (sternal margin).

Patient controlled epidural analgesia (PCEA):

- With background infusion – Infusion 5–8 ml/h; bolus 5 ml bupivacaine 0.1% + fentanyl 2 μg/ml OR ropivacaine 0.2%. Lock-out time 20 minutes.
- Without background infusion – Bolus 5 ml bupivacaine 0.1% + fentanyl 2 μg/ml OR ropivacaine 0.2%. Lock-out time 15 minutes.

---

discomfort occurs, and to the midwife that the dose must be given as soon as requested. The commonest cause of pain with a previously working epidural is delay in top-up administration. The practice of letting epidurals wear off for second stage labour is not acceptable.

Complications of epidural analgesia

- Hypotension. This should always be avoided in obstetric practice, as placental perfusion is proportional to maternal blood pressure. Ensure that there is no aortocaval compression (move patient onto her side or use a wedge) and apply at least 40 per cent oxygen. If there is no response to an initial fluid bolus of 300–500 ml, give ephedrine 3–6 mg, titrated to effect. Do not

---

Box 5.5. Effects of regional analgesia on the mother and fetus

- Delivery – evidence with low-dose epidurals appears to indicate that they increase the likelihood of an instrumental delivery but not of Caesarean section. The controversy in this area continues, as it is very difficult to allow for the fact that those labouring women who are heading for an instrumental delivery are more likely to request or be offered regional analgesia in labour when interpreting raw population data.
- Uterine function – this is not affected by regional analgesia provided hypotension or aortocaval compression is avoided. Indeed, in women with incoordinate or dysfunctional uterine contraction the drop in circulating catecholamine levels brought on with complete pain relief often improves the effectiveness of contractions.
- Uterine blood flow – this is not reduced in normal mothers, and may increase after epidural blockade in pre-eclamptic patients (see Chapter 3 for further details).

---

use an α-agonist, as these agents worsen already compromised placental perfusion.
- Dural puncture. This occurs in 0.5–1.0 per cent of epidurals. By far the largest risk factor is an inexperienced anaesthetist. Dural puncture is not of itself a problem, as long as it is noticed and an undiagnosed spinal catheter is not sited (see above – test doses). However, 30–50 per cent of mothers with Tuohy needle punctures go on to get a post dural puncture headache. These are characterized by an onset on the first postnatal day and may be very debilitating. Treatment is discussed in Box 5.7. Untreated, the headache usually eases between the fifth and tenth postnatal days, although cases have been reported of patients remaining symptomatic for over 9 months. In patients where dural puncture is known to have occurred, two analgesic options exist. A spinal catheter can be passed and 1 ml top-ups of low-dose mixture given as required by the anaesthetist. Alternatively, the epidural can be re-sited at another level. In all cases the patient should be informed of the tap, and actively followed up to assess for headache. Evidence now suggests that the use of spinal catheters does not decrease headache rates in known dural punctures.
- Failed or inadequate block – see above.
- 'Massive' spinal. This occurs when an epidural dose of local anaesthetic is given into the CSF due to inadvertent and

---

Box 5.6. Sorting out the problem epidural

- Missed segment – this has become a much less common problem since the routine addition of opioids to epidural mixtures. The most effective solution is to lie the patient on her unblocked side, withdraw the epidural catheter so that only 2–3 cm remains in the space, and give 10 ml bupivacaine 0.1% ± fentanyl 50 μg. Leave the patient lying for at least 5 minutes. If this fails, consider replacing the epidural.
- Unilateral block – rarely, complete block is achieved on one side of the patient with no effect on the other. The catheter tip travelling anteriorly and deflecting from fibrous strands running from the dura to the posterior longitudinal ligament causes this. Withdrawing the catheter so that 3 cm maximally remains in the space and giving another dose usually rectifies the problem. If it doesn't, replace the catheter but warn the patient that the problem may recur – a small proportion of the population have an anterior septum in the epidural space as a variant of normal anatomy.
- Sacral/ rectal pain – this is usually associated with a posterior fetal occiput and prolonged labour with poorly coordinated contractions. The pain is severe and unremitting even when the contraction pain is completely removed. Fentanyl is effective in reducing this, so 8–10 ml bupivacaine 0.1% + fentanyl 50 μg with the mother sitting upright for 10 minutes afterwards usually brings swift relief.

---

unrecognized catheter misplacement. Clinically, there is a rapid ascent of block associated with hypotension and, if the mixture reaches the brainstem, apnoea. Summon help as soon as the diagnosis is suspected. Treatment is supportive – ventilation, intravenous fluids and ephedrine as required. Continuous fetal monitoring is mandatory, and a low threshold should exist for urgent Caesarean section to deliver the baby.

- Local anaesthetic toxicity – inadvertent intravenous administration. Occasionally, the catheter may be placed with its tip inside an epidural vein. The symptoms of local anaesthetic toxicity are dose related, and are summarized in Box 5.8. Again, summon help early. Treatment is supportive. The doses of local anaesthetic used in low-dose epidurals are not sufficient to cause cardiac effects in healthy mothers. However, when infusions are used this can occur, and ventricular fibrillation secondary to bupivacaine toxicity is very resistant to treatment. For this reason ropivacaine and, more recently, laevo-bupivacaine are being marketed as safer, as they have better toxic side effect profiles.

Box 5.7. Post dural puncture headache (PDPH)

- Diagnosis: history of dural tap (80 per cent); occipital headache with postural component, relieved by lying down, abdominal compression and Valsalva manoeuvre; associated nausea, vomiting and meningism.
- Differential diagnoses of post delivery headache: PDPH, pre-eclamptic headache, subdural or subarachnoid haemorrhage, simple tension or migraine headache, meningitis and cortical vein thrombosis.
- Conservative treatment: keep the patient well hydrated, and well analgesed with codeine, paracetamol and NSAIDs. Lie her flat.
- Aggressive treatment: for those with severe symptoms and a clear-cut diagnosis, there is no point in waiting 24–48 hours to see if the pain settles. A blood patch is needed. This is the injection of up to 20 ml of autologous blood into the epidural space to form a fibrin plug over the leak. A senior anaesthetist should perform this after informed written consent. The patient must be afebrile, and blood from the same sample should be sent for culture. Both sample collection and epidural should be performed under conditions of strict asepsis. The patient should be told to remain as horizontal as possible for several hours post-injection. Ninety-five per cent PDPH are relieved by 6 hours post-procedure.
- Other treatment: an epidural saline bolus (30 ml down the catheter at the end of labour) or infusion (500 ml over 24 hours) is said by proponents to decrease the need for a blood patch. Evidence for this is individual rather than in clear-cut randomized controlled trials.

- Subdural blockade. This is very rare, and is only achievable by accident. In this case, the epidural catheter is passed through the dura but not through the arachnoid mater. The block gained is usually a very extensive purely sensory blockade (often extending as high as $C_{2/3}$) that achieves maximal spread 40 minutes post-injection. Haemodynamic problems are rare, and the block recedes over the following hour.
- Infection. The risk of meningitis (or encephalitis if the dura is breached) is very low, and decreases further with the use of full asepsis, disposable equipment and sterile drugs and administration techniques. Treatment is microbiologically guided. Full clinical neurological assessment and urgent MRI scan are indicated to assess for spinal abscess formation, and surgical drainage is required urgently once the diagnosis is confirmed.
- Nerve/spinal damage. Spinal cord damage should not occur, as all obstetric epidurals are placed at a vertebral level below the

---

Box 5.8. Local anaesthetic toxicity

The following are sequential eects with increasing plasma concentration (due to membrane stabilizing properties):

- Peri-oral tingling and numbness.
- Light-headedness.
- Agitation, tremor.
- Unconsciousness and/or convulsions.
- Hypotension.
- Cardiac arrhythmias, including ventricular fibrillation.

---

cord. Direct nerve trauma is a rare complication, but when suspicions are aroused from the history, conduction studies provide a clear answer. Never inject local anaesthetic if a patient complains of deep back or leg pain. Most of the numb patches blamed on anaesthetists are entirely unrelated to epidural analgesia, and reflect a lack of understanding of dermatomal patterns. All patients referred as such should be fully assessed, and the site and spinal level of numbness documented. Numbness in the lower leg and 'saddle' area is particularly associated with forceps delivery-related neuropraxia. Any patient with genuine neurological deficit thought to be related to an epidural or spinal procedure, especially if worsening or involving motor or autonomic function changes, needs urgent spinal MRI or contrast-enhanced CT to exclude spinal haematoma. Urgent neurosurgical review may be required, with a view to decompression and haematoma evacuation.

- Pruritus. This is associated with the opioid content of the epidural mixture. It usually settles after a short time, but if it is severe or persistent repeated 10–20 mg bolus doses of propofol intravenously might help. Chlorpheniramine 10 mg i.m. or i.v. may also help, and has anxiolytic effects.

Other complications, including nausea, vomiting and shivering, can be treated as appropriate, provided that potentially serious underlying causes such as hypotension and hypoxia are ruled out first.

The combined spinal-epidural

The combined spinal-epidural (CSE) was introduced in the late 1980s as the solution to all the shortcomings of the epidural. The introduction into widespread practice of low-dose epidurals has rendered many of its purported advantages irrelevant, but this is still a useful technique. The major advantages and disadvantages are summarized in Box 5.9. Most CSEs are sited using a 'needle-through-needle' technique, but 'needle-beside needle' and 'different interspaces' techniques are also used.

In the 'needle-through-needle' technique, the Tuohy needle is sited in the extradural space as usual. A long 25–27G pencil-tip spinal needle is passed down the Tuohy and through the dura, and CSF is aspirated to confirm placement. A spinal starter is given (typically bupivacaine 2.5 mg plus fentanyl 25 µg), CSF is re-aspirated to ensure the needle has not moved, and then the spinal needle is removed and the catheter passed as normal.

The complications of the CSE are as for the epidural.

Second stage analgesia

Mothers who request epidural analgesia should only be denied this if one of the contraindications listed above is present. The second stage of labour is not a contraindication!

If analgesia is required for a ventouse or forceps delivery, several factors need to be assessed quickly. The suggested response to each is summarized in Box 5.10. The same contraindications to regional anaesthesia apply as for labour. These procedures often occur in a

---

Box 5.9. Combined spinal-epidurals – advantages and disadvantages in labour

Advantages:
- Faster onset of analgesia (this is an area of intense debate – it is claimed to be true by proponents of the CSE but has not been proven in the authors' opinion).
- Better perineal analgesia.
- Lower incidence of missed segments (claimed to be true, but again unproven).

Disadvantages:
- Breaching the dura unnecessarily, giving increased PDPH and infection risk.
- Higher cost.
- Higher incidence of proprioceptive impairment (may affect patient's ability to mobilize).

Box 5.10 Analgesia for instrumental delivery

- High risk of proceeding to LSCS, epidural previously sited: the patient needs a block that will cover both procedures. Epidural top-up: lignocaine 1.5–2% 15 ml epinephrine 1 : 200 000 fentanyl 50–100 µg.
- High risk of proceeding to LSCS, no epidural in situ: a fast block with the facility to extend is ideal. Spinal±CSE: bupivacaine 0.25% 2.5 ml plus fentanyl 25 µg.
- Low risk of proceeding to LSCS, epidural previously sited: a lower block is needed. Epidural top-up: lignocaine 1.5% 10 ml epinephrine 1 : 200 000 fentanyl 50–100 µg.
- Low risk of proceeding to LSCS, no epidural in situ: a spinal saddle block is ideal. Spinal: 1.5 ml heavy bupivacaine 0.5%, keep patient sitting upright for 1 minute then lie down.

---

separate area, but full monitoring and intravenous access are still required. This usually involves the establishment of a dense block in a patient going into the lithotomy position, so it is vital to be aware of the risks of aortocaval compression and insist on a wedge, table tilt or manual uterine displacement as appropriate.

6

Analgesia for labour II: other analgesic methods

Childbirth and the associated pain that goes with it has become an increasingly controversial area of discussion over the last 20 years. The predominant medical attitude of '...you wouldn't have a tooth out without local if you could avoid it so why have a baby without proper pain relief...' has often been at odds with the view of many women's groups that natural childbirth is vital and essential to maternal and fetal well being, and that all interventions are by their very nature wrong. These polarized views are less common today, with a greater emphasis on providing informed choice for the labouring woman. It is now a central role of the obstetric anaesthetist to act as an advisor and information resource on all available analgesic options. This chapter covers all the main forms of non-regional analgesia used in the UK in labouring women.

Pain in labour

The pain associated with childbirth is of far too complex aetiology to be considered purely in terms of nerve supply. The descriptions given by parturients of their pain vary hugely depending on psychological, social and organizational factors, including time of questioning, prenatal expectations, level of staff support and outcome of the labour. The relevant nerve supplies are discussed in more detail in Chapter 5. The success or failure of non-epidural based analgesia is also difficult to quantify, as pain reduction rather than complete relief is the best outcome achievable. However, this is perfectly acceptable to many women, and the likelihood of successful analgesia increases in those who understand their chosen method and more so in those who have used that method in previous labours. The features of an ideal labour analgesic are listed in Box 6.1.

Box 6.1. Properties of an ideal analgesic for labour

- Provides complete analgesia with rapid onset and offset.
- Simple to initiate.
- Non-invasive.
- Non-cumulative.
- Not metabolized.
- No harmful sequelae to use.
- No maternal or fetal side effects.
- No motor or sensory alterations, or central sedative effects.
- No effect on progression of labour.
- No anaphylactic risk.
- No drug interactions.
- Inexpensive.
- Can be used by all women irrespective of health.

Pharmacological analgesia in labour

Inhalational analgesia – Entonox

Entonox (50 per cent nitrous oxide in oxygen) has been widely used as an inhalational analgesic during labour since its introduction into widespread usage during the 1960s, and it is the commonest analgesic used in labour in the UK today. The gases are stable when mixed in the cylinder unless the temperature falls to below $-6°C$, when they separate, causing the nitrous oxide to fall to the dependent part of the cylinder (the Poynting effect). The ensuing inhaled mixture is thus initially almost pure oxygen, providing no analgesia, and later becomes an anaesthetic, hypoxic, nitrous oxide-rich gas. Cylinders that have been stored in the cold should therefore be assumed to have separated. Prior to use, these should either be subsequently stored at over $10°C$ for at least 24 hours, or placed in a body temperature water bath for 5 minutes. They should then be inverted three times to ensure mixing of the contents.

Entonox is delivered to the patient via a two-stage reducing and on-demand valve, which fits directly on to the cylinder and uses the pin index agent specificity system. A small negative pressure is all that is required to activate a high gas flow from the cylinder. Delivery is through a facemask or mouthpiece, and the mixture is self-administered so that, in the event of the mother becoming drowsy, the delivery system is released before unconsciousness occurs.

The technique of inhalational analgesia must be taught so that maximum benefit is obtained. This should ideally happen in antenatal classes, but often needs to be explained to the mother when she arrives in labour. Nitrous oxide has a low blood/gas solubility, and so lung–blood–brain equilibration is rapid. Even so, Entonox needs to be inhaled for about 45 seconds before the maximum analgesic effect is obtained. Thus, deep inhalation must start when the onset of the contraction is first felt, rather than 20–30 seconds later when the pain starts. This slow, deep breathing pattern should be continued right through the contraction.

Studies have indicated that about half the women who try Entonox will have adequate analgesia (a rate twice that of those given pethidine alone), but about a quarter find it no help at all.

The advantages and disadvantages of Entonox are listed in Box 6.2.

Volatile anaesthetics ± Entonox
Throughout the history of anaesthesia inhalational agents such as chloroform, ether and methoxyflurane have been used in childbirth either as stand-alone analgesics or in combination with Entonox. Papers have recently been published regarding low concentrations

---

Box 6.2. Advantages and disadvantages of Entonox for analgesia in labour

Advantages:
- Safe to mother and fetus.
- 'Low tech' – needs no expert staff or specialized equipment.
- Fast onset and offset of effect.
- Inexpensive.
- Can be used in conjunction with all other forms of analgesia used in labour.

Disadvantages:
- Inadequate analgesia in high proportion of users.
- Bulky, heavy cylinders to be moved about.
- Maternal cooperation and competence needed for effective use.
- Slight concerns still exist over protracted use in labour increasing risk of nitrous oxide-mediated methionine synthetase inhibition, folate metabolism and DNA synthesis.

of isoflurane or sevoflurane added to Entonox. These mixtures show some increase in analgesic efficacy over Entonox alone, but have yet to catch on in widespread practice.

Opioids – Pethidine
Intramuscular pethidine is the most common opioid used in labour, and can be given in doses of 50–150 mg by unsupervised midwives. At this dose the analgesic effects should become apparent after 10–15 minutes and last for about 3 hours. The usual dose used is 100 mg, and research has shown this dose is ineffective as the sole analgesic in 60–75 per cent of patients. Intravenous pethidine via a patient-controlled analgesia (PCA) pump provides much better analgesia, but almost double the amount is used compared to nurse-controlled administration.

Pethidine causes nausea and vomiting in up to 50 per cent of mothers, and may also produce sedation sufficient to impair co-operation during labour and delivery and alter long-term memory of the process. The fetal effects of opioids during labour are discussed fully in Chapter 3, but include respiratory depression if delivery is within 1–2 hours of administration, and later (3–6 hours post-administration) depression of Apgar and neurobehavioural scores. This later effect is thought to be due to toxic effects of norpethidine. The advantages and disadvantages of pethidine are summarized in Box 6.3.

Other opioids
Morphine is rarely used in labour because of its long duration of action. Partial opioid agonists (nalbuphine, pentazocine, butorphanol) have been used in place of pethidine with little benefit and an increased incidence of nausea, vomiting and dysphoria in some cases.

Given the problems associated with opioid use in labour, together with the poor analgesia provided, their role is increasingly being questioned. The recent development of the ultra-short acting opioid remifentanil has led to some revived interest in PCA analgesia. This is used in a similar way to Entonox in those cases where epidural analgesia is contraindicated, not possible or not wanted. This is still at an experimental stage, but may offer a future role for opioids in labour.

Box 6.3. Advantages and disadvantages of intramuscular pethidine analgesia in labour

Advantages:
- Anxiolytic effect.
- Does not require medical input.
- Inexpensive.

Disadvantages:
- Poor analgesia.
- Maternal side effects – nausea, vomiting, sedation, risk of respiratory depression.
- Fetal side effects – loss of beat-to-beat variability, depression of Apgar and neurobehavioural scores, risk of respiratory depression.

Non-pharmacological analgesia in labour

Many varieties of non-pharmacological analgesia have been used over the centuries to ease the pain of labour, ranging from deep breathing patterns to transcendental meditation. Psychoprophylaxis for labour at its most basic level is undeniably a good idea, as a mother who is informed and prepared for what lies ahead will be much less anxious and thus experience less pain amplification during contractions. However, some practitioners in this sector claim that, with proper use of breathing and relaxation exercises, the pain of labour can be abolished. This is an appealing assertion, and those mothers who believe it are often very upset when reality differs from the preconception.

This section covers the more accepted and common techniques employed.

Transcutaneous electrical nerve stimulation

This method follows the gate theory of pain, and uses low voltage electrical stimulation either side of the lower thoracic spine to attempt to prevent nociceptive signals ascending the cord. Whilst its efficacy in the later stages of labour and delivery is low, many women find transcutaneous electrical nerve stimulation (TENS) useful in early labour and it is often used at home prior to admission to the obstetric unit. The device lets the mother adjust the level of stimulation, and this element of self-control also increases patient satisfaction. Machines are small, easily portable, battery powered, and can be rented or purchased inexpensively from high street chemists or groups such as the National Childbirth Trust.

Hypnosis

Hypnosis carries obvious advantages in terms of complete drug avoidance for mother and child. However, only a small proportion of labouring women can be hypnotized to a level where effective analgesia is produced, and the hypnotist must be present throughout labour.

Acupuncture

This has not been shown in the UK to be of any benefit in labour. However, it is reportedly used to great effect in mainland China and the Far East.

Aromatherapy, crystal power and other 'New Age' treatments

These are of no clinical benefit, although they may psychologically assist the mother if she believes that they will help. These treatments are unlikely to be harmful, so if a mother wants to try it she should not be stopped!

7

Regional anaesthesia for Caesarean section

Traditionally, Caesarean section has been classified as either elective or emergency. These terms are inadequate and vague, elective meaning scheduled surgery and all other cases being classed as emergency. The difficulty with emergency as a classification is that the degree of urgency is open to varying degrees of interpretation. True maternal or fetal life-threatening situations are rare but of great importance, and in these cases correct decision making from both obstetricians and anaesthetists is paramount. Attempts to improve the definition have led to the proposed classification shown in Box 7.1.

It is important for the anaesthetist to remain in control of the section at all times, irrespective of the degree of urgency. It is easy, especially in the emergency situation, to feel pressurized by obstetricians and patients to start surgery before effective analgesia has occurred. Obstetricians can only start when the anaesthetist is confident with the height and intensity of the block.

General preoperative measures

General measures (Box 7.2) must also include the assessment of a patient who may have a general anaesthetic. It is important to remember that airway anatomy can alter throughout labour, and

---

Box 7.1. Classification of urgency of Caesarean section

Grade 1/Emergency	Immediate threat to maternal or fetal life
Grade 2/Urgent	Maternal or fetal compromise that is not immediately life threatening
Grade 3/Scheduled	Needing early delivery, no maternal or fetal compromise
Grade 4/Elective	At a time chosen to suit the operative team and the mother

---

Box 7.2. General measures prior to Caesarean section under regional anaesthesia

- Consent.
- Explanation.
- Trained anaesthetic assistant (mandatory).
- Antacid therapy.
- Starvation.
- Indwelling intravenous cannula.
- Left lateral tilt of 5° – avoid aortocaval compression.
- Preparation and assessment for potential general anaesthetic conversion.

---

that a previous assessment of easy intubation may change over 12 hours. A small number of regional anaesthetics need to be converted to general anaesthesia because of anaesthetic failure, obstetric complications or maternal request.

Antacid therapy is given to all Caesarean section patients irrespective of the type of anaesthesia used. Sodium citrate is the alkali of choice as it is non-particulate and, if aspirated, has not been implicated as a factor in the development of Mendelson's syndrome. Magnesium hydroxide was used in the past, but if aspirated was implicated as causative of aspiration pneumonitis because of its particulate nature. It is claimed that sodium citrate is effective at raising the gastric contents to above pH 2.5 if given less than 15 minutes prior to surgery. In the emergency situation often it is only possible to neutralize the stomach contents. A typical regimen is shown in Box 7.3.

The benefits of allowing women to eat and drink in labour are humanitarian rather than medical. Calorific intake has not yet been shown to be of any great maternal or fetal benefit. A starved patient presents less of an anaesthetic challenge than one with a full stomach, although all obstetric patients must be regarded as at risk of aspiration. Patients for elective obstetric procedures are normally starved for 6 hours.

General intraoperative measures

Most anaesthetists routinely provide 40 per cent oxygen via an appropriate device such as a Hudson mask at least until the baby is delivered. There is little evidence that this is beneficial, and often mothers find the mask very uncomfortable to tolerate. Caesarean

---

Box 7.3. Typical antacid regimens for patients undergoing Caesarean section

---

- Elective section – 12 hours preoperatively (often night before), oral ranitidine 150 mg; 2 hours preoperatively, oral ranitidine 150 mg + metoclopramide 10 mg. Within 15 minutes of the surgery, oral sodium citrate 0.3 M, 30 ml.
- Emergency section – within 15 minutes of surgery, oral sodium citrate 0.3 M, 30 ml. Intravenous metoclopramide 10 mg + intravenous ranitidine 50 mg may be given at the anaesthetist's discretion.
- At-risk patients in labour – nil by mouth, oral ranitidine 150 mg 8-hourly at the discretion of the anaesthetist, midwife or obstetrician.
- Patients receiving pethidine in labour – may be given intramuscular metoclopramide 10 mg with the first dose, but are not routinely considered at risk.

---

section carries the risk of sepsis and endometritis, and for this reason antibiotics are routinely given. It is customary to give them after the birth of the baby, and not to prepare them until this time so as to avoid potential antibiotic–thiopentone confusion. Normally intravenous cefuroxime 1.5 g is given, but some units use intravenous co-amoxiclav 1.2 g. In cases of suspected penicillin sensitivity, erythromycin 500 mg is used.

Intravenous oxytocin 5–10 iu is given after the delivery of the baby to aid uterine contraction and prevent blood loss. It is vital not to give it before delivery; it can easily be given in error before the birth of a second twin in a multiple birth. It is sensible practice, therefore, to draw it up after the delivery of the baby(ies), as this reduces the risk of error. Uterine contraction asphyxiates the fetus and makes delivery in Caesarean section almost impossible. Oxytocin has also been given in error in place of suxamethonium for intubation. Keeping the antibiotics and other non-anaesthetic drugs in separate containers away from anaesthetic induction agents and relaxants minimizes the chance of wrongful administration. Occasionally the obstetrician asks for a syntocinon infusion if the uterus is slow to contract down. This can be prepared as 40 iu diluted in 500 ml of normal saline and given over 4 hours. It is also easy to give intravenous drugs down the epidural catheter in error, and this must also be avoided!

Contraindications

The contraindications to regional anaesthesia for Caesarean section are as for any regional procedure – patient refusal, cardiovascular instability, coagulopathy, allergy and sepsis. Coagulopathy can occur in pre-eclampsia, intrauterine death, and placental abruption. Occasionally, idiopathic thrombocytopenia of pregnancy can occur. Most people perform regional anaesthesia for Caesarean section with a platelet count of $80 \times 10^9/l$ where there is not a continuous downward trend in the count.

Choice of technique

Practically, there are only three choices available, although direct infiltration with local anaesthetic is still mentioned. These are epidural, spinal, or combined spinal-epidural (CSE) anaesthesia. The advantages and disadvantages of the epidural and spinal techniques are shown in Boxes 7.4 and 7.5 respectively.

Epidural anaesthesia for Caesarean section is used commonly when an existing catheter for use as labour analgesia is in place or when there is a medical indication, such as pre-existing cardiac disease, for a carefully controlled incremental dosage. Spinal or combined spinal-epidural anaesthesia is chosen by many for both elective and emergency surgery.

The combined spinal-epidural technique was designed to maximize the benefits of both techniques and minimize the disadvantages. It succeeds in the main, but is expensive. The epidural catheter can be used to extend or prolong the spinal block, and is often used to provide postoperative analgesia.

Box 7.4. Advantages and disadvantages of epidural anaesthesia for Caesarean section

Advantages:
- Easy to extend existing block.
- No dural puncture.
- Can be extended slowly for greater cardiovascular stability.
- Less need for large intravenous pre-loading.
- Postoperative analgesia can be provided via the catheter.
- Less equipment and cheaper than other methods.

Disadvantages:
- Slow onset.
- Block can be patchy with missed segments.
- Can be unpredictable in spread.

Box 7.5. Advantages and disadvantages of spinal anaesthesia for Caesarean section

Advantages:

- Normally quick to perform.
- Rapid speed of onset.
- Little patient discomfort experienced intraoperatively.
- Relatively inexpensive when compared to other techniques.

Disadvantages:

- Large intravenous pre-loading often needed, hypotension more common.
- Single-shot technique.
- Unpredictable time duration of block.
- Wears off rapidly.
- Dural puncture (risk of infection and headache increased).

What to tell the patient

Consent, risks and benefits of the technique should have been explained to the patient before she arrives in the theatre. The risk of post dural puncture headache should again be mentioned. The authors' practice is to explain every part of the procedure as it is performed, as patients are often anxious about having procedures carried out that they cannot see. The intravenous cannula should be inserted using local anaesthetic. After the procedure has been performed, it is sensible practice to remind the patient that the surgeon will not be allowed to start until the block has been checked and is proven to be adequate. The patient should also be told that she will go numb up to her chest. She should inform the anaesthetist if her hands start to tingle (high block), or if she feels light-headed, dizzy or nauseated, as these are signs of a drop in blood pressure and will need to be treated. Patients are aware of hypotension often before it is apparent on the non-invasive blood pressure monitoring device. In the authors' experience, nausea and vomiting are nearly always due to hypotension irrespective of cuff blood pressure readings, and settle with incremental ephedrine 3–6 mg.

Technique

A strict aseptic technique should be used. This means gloves, gown, hat and mask.

The position of the patient for the block is often discussed. Normally regional anaesthesia is performed in the sitting position with the patient's feet on a stool and the patient curved forwards over a pillow in an attempt to flex the lumbar spine. Some anaesthetists favour the right lateral position and claim that if a spinal block is being performed, the right side is blocked immediately from gravitational effects and then the left side is effectively blocked when the patient is placed in the left lateral tilt position. Other practitioners place the patient in the left lateral position and then turn her onto a left lateral tilt. They report that although the block is slightly slower to be effective on the right side, effective analgesia can be achieved without tilting the patient onto the right (aortocaval compression). Occasionally it is impossible to site a block due to bony obstruction. A change of patient position or a different practitioner normally allows for the successful placement of the catheter or needle. It is no shame to be unable to insert an epidural – it happens to everyone.

Dose regimens for Caesarean section

There is a huge variety of drug regimens that are used successfully. Normally anaesthetists add opiate such as fentanyl or diamorphine (fat-soluble) to enhance the speed of onset, improve the quality of analgesia, prolong the duration of the block, and enhance the quality of postoperative analgesia. The potential side effects of drowsiness, vomiting, nausea, respiratory depression and itching have to be balanced against the benefits. Suitable doses are shown in Box 7.6.

How much solution is required to top up an existing labour epidural?

This is variable, and it is claimed that as little as 8 ml may be needed when topping up a regional block that has just been inserted and the initial labour dose given. Sometimes an incremental dose of up to 20 ml is necessary. Some practitioners add 1 ml bicarbonate 8.4% to the epidural top-up mixture to alkalinize it and hasten the speed of onset of the block, but the authors find this unnecessary. Epinephrine lowers the potentially toxic dose of lignocaine that can be given, but carries with it the potential of a rare spinal artery spasm; the authors use it. The more complicated the mixture, the more likelihood there is of making a drug mistake – normal saline can be confused with lignocaine, and epinephrine 1 : 1000 can be confused with atropine.

Box 7.6. Suitable drug dosages for Caesarean section

- Epidural anaesthesia: 0.5% plain bupivacaine, 2% lignocaine with 1:200000 epinephrine, or a combination of 2% lignocaine + 0.5% bupivacaine. Incremental dosage is used to 20–25 ml in total. Fentanyl 50–100 µg may be added to these solutions.
- Spinal/CSE anaesthesia: 2.5 ml 0.5% heavy bupivacaine ± 25 µg fentanyl (or ± 0.25 µg diamorphine).

Fluid management

Most anaesthetists use Hartmann's solution for fluid management. For spinal anaesthesia in a healthy patient, normally 1 l can be given during block insertion, and often a second litre is given during the operation. Some practitioners pre-load with gelatin on the principle that intravascular compartment expansion is needed in an attempt to counteract the relative hypovolaemia secondary to the sympathetic blockade and vasodilation that occurs. The hypotension with spinal anaesthesia can be rapid and profound. For epidural analgesia, the block is slower in onset and less of a pre-load is needed. Most give about half a litre. A large-bore cannula must be sited and well secured prior to the start of the block; this then ensures safety if surgery becomes complicated.

Monitoring the patient, the height of the block and when to start

The patient is normally given oxygen 40 per cent (4 l/min) via an appropriate mask (e.g. Hudson) after being placed in the left lateral tilt position. The pulse oximeter, electrocardiograph and non-invasive blood pressure monitor are attached prior to block insertion. It is sensible to take the blood pressure every 3 minutes after siting the block whilst watching for hypotension. The height of the block needs to be assessed. This is normally done using ethyl chloride spray, which is cold – patients cannot differentiate between temperature once the block is established. The block needs to ascend to about the level of the T_4 dermatome bilaterally (nipple level), and descend to the sacral nerve roots (the perineum). Patients should not experience the pain of urinary catheterization; this is an indication that the sacral roots are blocked. Normally the patient is unable to lift her legs when the block is adequate. With a spinal anaesthetic the onset time can be as short as 5 minutes, but with a slowly topped-up epidural it may take 30 minutes to be effective. The anaesthetic is now ready and the wait for the obstetricians can begin!

Intraoperative problems

Normally Caesarean sections are uneventful, but even the most experienced anaesthetist finds that difficulties can arise due to surgery, the anaesthetic, or because the patient cannot cope. Surgery should not be 'rough', and everyone in theatre should be aware that the patient and her partner are not deaf. If the block is good, the uterus may be 'delivered' without any physiological abnormality or maternal discomfort.

Hypotension

Hypotension is best prevented. Mothers feel ill and vomit with hypotension. Often they feel anxious and restless when this occurs. An adequate pre-load in parturients who are systemically well is in the order of 1 l. Ensure that a left lateral tilt is in place to prevent aortocaval compression. The uterus can also be manually displaced to the left if needed. Ephedrine is the sympathomimetic drug of choice, as it does not cause vasoconstriction in the placenta. Most practitioners have a low threshold for giving 6 mg bolus doses, and often up to 60 mg is needed. Some anaesthetists give less of a pre-load and place 30 mg in the litre of Hartmann's solution, but the authors don't use this as it gives the mothers an unacceptable tachycardia.

Nausea and vomiting

Nausea and vomiting is often due to hypotension, which should be treated first. Occasionally it is due to visceral traction and can be treated with intravenous metoclopramide 10 mg. Intravenous ondansetron 4–8 mg may be used, but it is worth noting that the British National Formulary states that it is cautioned in pregnancy and breast-feeding.

High block

As nearly all anaesthetists use heavy bupivacaine as the drug of choice, it seems sensible to place the patient head-up if she complains of tingling or weakness in the arms or hands. The authors prefer to use pillows under the patient's head to prevent high spread. If a very high block develops, respiratory embarrassment will ensue and the patient will need to be anaesthetized and ventilated until the block has worn off. It often takes about 10–20 minutes for a high block to recede to an acceptable height.

Dysrhythmias

Dysrhythmias are not uncommon during Caesarean section. Commonly, the tachycardia of anxiety in the mother is replaced by a bradycardia as the block ascends and blocks the sympathomimetic cardiac accelerator fibres. A relative bradycardia is a sign that the block is working. Ectopic beats of all varieties have been reported, and are not associated with any morbidity. They resolve spontaneously in the main and their aetiology is unclear. Myocardial ischaemia has been suggested because, rarely, ST segment elevation occurs on the electrocardiograph, but this is unlikely. Dysrhythmias are probably multifactorial, with the effects of hypotension and surgical manipulation being most likely.

Pruritus

Patients complain of itching due to the spinal or epidural opiates that they have been given. No treatment is particularly effective, so mothers need to be reassured that this is not serious and will settle quickly. The recently suggested regimen of repeated intravenous propofol 10 mg bolus doses can be helpful in some cases. Some authors advise naloxone in 100–200 µg bolus doses to effect.

Substernal and epigastric discomfort

Following delivery of the baby, mothers often complain of epigastric or substernal ache, described as 'a stitch' or a feeling of being 'winded'. This is due to the surgery, and is not clinically significant. Continued reassurance that it will settle quickly and is not serious is all that is required. Once peritoneal traction and swabbing stops, the sensation passes.

Pain

It is important that the anaesthetist makes the right judgement with respect to the amount of discomfort that the patient is feeling. Some discomfort is to be expected when the baby is being delivered, as there is quite a lot of pressure exerted on the upper abdomen. This can be disconcerting if the mother is not expecting it. Many surgeons wish to deliver the uterus outside the abdominal cavity after delivery to aid access for uterine closure. This can cause discomfort that settles once the uterus is replaced within the abdomen. If there is significant pain from the surgery (missed segment, inadequate block), action must be taken promptly. A decision must be made as to whether the pain can be managed under augmented regional anaesthesia or whether general anaesthesia is required. Methods of augmentation include Entonox, intravenous opoids (such as fentanyl in 10–25 µg bolus doses) titrated to effect, or topping up the epidural with 5–10 ml of lignocaine 2% with fentanyl 50 µg whilst surgery is stopped. Patient anxiety is always an important factor, and constant communication between the anaesthetist and the patient is vital at this time.

Conversion to general anaesthesia

Inducing general anaesthesia during surgery is not easy. It is difficult to anaesthetize safely with a patient 'draped' half way through an operation, and with a potential degree of haemodynamic compromise from regional anaesthesia. This said, it sometimes has to be done, but the same care and preparation must be exercised as for any other rapid sequence induction. Obstetricians may exert pressure to 'convert' if the patient is vocal in her discomfort, but the anaesthetist must not be influenced by this.

It is vital that the patient is in the correct position for intubation. In regional anaesthesia, the neck is often flexed upwards and the head of the operating table raised. This must be manipulated to be in the best position for intubation prior to anaesthetic induction. Full pre-oxygenation must occur and the drapes must be moved so that adequate access to the neck is possible. Surgery must be halted whilst anaesthesia is induced, and it must be made clear that this may only restart when the anaesthetist says so.

Note taking

Documentation is important in these increasingly litigious days, especially in the emergency situation. Delays in delivery are often blamed erroneously on the anaesthetist. It is therefore recommended that the anaesthetist notes the following times: notification of emergency Caesarean section; arrival of the patient on the table; the time the block was deemed ready for surgery to start; the time surgery started; and the time of delivery. An upper limit of 15 minutes from the decision to operate until delivery is a gold standard that all units should aim for in the emergency situation.

All drugs and fluids given must be noted correctly in both dose and time, and minimum monitoring observations must be recorded every 5 minutes (pulse, blood pressure and oxygen saturation). Block height pre-incision is important, as well as the technique used and complications encountered. If data are recorded in retrospect, state this on the chart. Where possible, a computerized data printout is a useful addition to hand-written notes.

Postoperative analgesia

Spinal analgesia alone can wear off quickly, and a variety of methods are available to assist with postoperative analgesic provision. Box 7.7 lists the common methods in use for an uncomplicated Caesarean section.

Prevention of thromboembolism

Pulmonary embolism is the major cause of maternal mortality in labour, and consideration of its prevention is still poor in the UK as a whole. Regional anaesthesia decreases the risk of deep vein

---

Box 7.7. Methods of postoperative analgesia suitable for Caesarean section

Intraoperative methods:

- Opioid addition: fentanyl 25 μg or diamorphine 0.25 mg to the spinal solution; or diamorphine 2.5–5.0 mg diluted in 10 ml normal saline through the epidural catheter at the end of the procedure.

Postoperative methods:

- Non-steroidal anti-inflammatory drugs (diclofenac 50–100 mg suppository at the end of the operation (with patient consent) to a maximum of 150 mg/day).
- Long-acting opioids (such as intramuscular morphine 0.15 mg/kg) at the end of the operation and 3–4-hourly thereafter, or intravenous morphine (1 mg bolus with a 5 minute lock-out time) via a PCA machine.
- Oral drugs such as mixtures of codeine phosphate 30 mg + paracetamol 500 mg in tablet form, with one or two being taken every 4 hours to a maximum of eight daily.
- Continuation of epidural analgesia by infusion or patient-controlled pump.

Box 7.8. Thromboembolism prevention in Caesarean section

All patients are admitted for bed rest to have TED stockings.

- Low risk patient (elective Caesarean section with early mobilization/hydration) – no special measures.
- Moderate risk patient (age >35 years, obesity (>80 kg), para four or more, gross varicose veins, concurrent infection, major systemic disease, pre-eclampsia) – TED stockings.
- High risk patient (three or more of above moderate risk factors OR extended surgery OR family history OR emergency Caesarean section) – TED stockings + low molecular weight heparin (dalteparin 2500 iu) until full mobilization.

---

thrombosis. Various units have different policies that are based on a Royal College of Obstetricians Working Party Report published in 1995. A typical policy is shown in Box 7.8.

These guidelines need to be assessed for each case. Low molecular weight heparin may increase the incidence of wound haematoma and the risk of epidural haematoma. The use of non-steroidal anti-inflammatory drugs may be contraindicated in patients with renal disease (including pre-eclampsia), asthma, or on anticoagulants. Delayed return of normal leg movement would be a cause for suspicion of an epidural haematoma in a patient who has had a Caesarean section.

8

General anaesthesia for Caesarean section

General anaesthesia, especially for emergency procedures, has always been a significant cause of maternal mortality. This has arisen mainly from the complications of intubation – hypoxia and aspiration. Therefore, current practice is aimed at avoiding general anaesthesia wherever possible. It is impossible always to avoid general anaesthesia, and often it is performed under the most difficult circumstances, such as severe placental abruption.

Airway
Intubation is often difficult and stressful for the anaesthetist. It is important to remember that airway assessment can change throughout labour, especially in patients who have pre-eclampsia. Pharyngeal wall oedema can alter the ease of intubation dramatically over a few hours, and asking for help prior to a potentially difficult intubation is sensible and may prove essential. Help for the solitary obstetric anaesthetist can be a long time arriving in an isolated maternity unit. The most important consideration, especially in patients who are undergoing emergency Caesarean section, is the decision regarding what course of action to take if intubation is not possible (see failed intubation). Vomiting on induction can occur in all women, particularly in those who have been given pethidine, have eaten recently or have aortocaval compression.

Management of anaesthesia
All equipment must be checked and suction equipment made available and positioned at the patient's head. Sodium citrate 0.3 M 30 ml should be given, and the patient positioned supine with a left lateral tilt. Full 3-minute 100 per cent pre-oxygenation must occur. It is easy to make a patient hypercarbic using a Mapleson D system if the rotameter flow rate isn't adequate. Often a flow rate of 10 l/min is needed through a tightly fitting

mask. The capnograph can be attached whilst pre-oxygenation is being carried out to ensure that normocarbia (P_aCO_2 of about 4 per cent in the term pregnant woman) is maintained. Anaesthesia should not commence without a trained anaesthetic nurse or operating department practitioner.

An induction dose of thiopentone is used with cricoid pressure being applied by an experienced, trained assistant. Suxamethonium is still the drug of choice for facilitating intubation as it has the fastest onset and offset. Cricoid pressure is removed after clinical and capnographic confirmation of correct tracheal tube placement. Difficulties with intubation arise because of incorrect patient head positioning, the patient's hair being tied back in a bun or ponytail (which interferes with neck extension), anaesthetic anxiety, intubation attempts before the relaxant has worked, difficulty in inserting the laryngoscope blade due to the patient's breasts or the anaesthetic assistant's hands, and incorrect cricoid pressure placement. Airway oedema may be present, and many anaesthetists routinely use a 7.0–7.5 mm ID endotracheal tube. Maintenance of anaesthesia is normally with 50 per cent nitrous oxide in oxygen with a suitable concentration of volatile agent (isoflurane or sevoflurane). Volatile agents relax the uterus, but this is not a major clinical problem and they must be given to prevent awareness. A FiO_2 of 0.5 is adequate for placental perfusion of oxygen. Following delivery of the baby the mother is given analgesia (intravenous morphine up to 20 mg), antibiotics and oxytocin. The muscle relaxant is reversed in routine fashion at the end of the operation, and the patient is extubated when fully awake with intact airway reflexes.

Potential problems
Drug errors
These will occur unless scrupulous care is taken and all drugs are carefully double-checked. It is easy to confuse the 20 ml syringe containing the antibiotic with that containing thiopentone. Oxytocin can be mixed up, when under pressure, with the 2 ml syringe containing suxamethonium. It is wise to have two trays; one for the induction agents and another for other drugs.

Awareness
Light general anaesthesia was once considered acceptable because the compromised fetus would be less affected by anaesthesia.

However, pain and awareness in anaesthesia are associated with poor placental perfusion, so they are undesirable from a physiological and humanitarian perspective. An adequate induction dose of anaesthetic should always be used and a volatile agent added. An agent-monitoring device is mandatory. Awareness causes enormous stress to the mother, and often it is not mentioned to the anaesthetist on the routine postoperative visit. The details emerge slowly, often via a trusted midwife or a relative. Psychiatric counselling is often needed, following careful discussion with the patient, and clinical risk management should take place to ensure the problem does not occur again.

Hypertensive response to intubation
This is not a great problem in healthy mothers. In mothers who are already hypertensive the response can be accentuated, and in these patients should be attenuated. This can be achieved with alfentanil 10–20 µg/kg but it may cause neonatal depression, and the paediatricians will need to be prewarned. Magnesium sulphate given intravenously in a dose of 40 mg/kg is also effective, but may potentiate neuromuscular blockade.

Recovery area
Many units have no recovery area, and patients are recovered in the operating theatre. Some midwives are trained recovery staff, but most are not and have little experience with dealing with the unconscious patient. Anaesthetists tend to recover the patients themselves and send them back to the delivery suite recovery room when they have fully awoken and are stable.

Failed intubation
Experience in general anaesthesia for Caesarean section is decreasing, and potentially trainees do it for the first time alone and in an emergency case. The incidence of failed intubation in this situation is claimed to be about 1 : 250–400, which is higher than in the general theatre environment, in which it is about 1 : 2500. The reasons for this are outlined above, and anaesthetic anxiety is a major factor. Overforceful and misplaced cricoid pressure impedes vision, as does poor head positioning and early intubation. Airway oedema and difficulty with laryngoscope blade insertion also occur. The important considerations are listed in Box 8.1. A proper airway assessment should take place prior to induction of anaesthesia.

Box 8.1. Important considerations for facilitating intubation

- Assess the airway carefully – Mallampatti, Patil, thyromental distance, jaw protrusion.
- Check intubation equipment and have the following available:

  Endotracheal tubes (range of sizes)
  Two working Macintosh laryngoscopes (standard and long blades)
  One short-handled Macintosh laryngoscope
  One Polio-bladed laryngoscope
  One McCoy laryngoscope
  Bougies
  Oral and nasal airways
  Laryngeal masks (sizes 3 and 4)
  Combitube
  Access to fibreoptic intubating laryngoscope
  Percutaneous cricothyroidotomy device and a circuit to connect it to an oxygen supply.

- Make a decision beforehand as to a plan of action if intubation is unsuccessful.
- Have intubation drugs close at hand.
- Make an early decision regarding whether intubation is possible, and abandon intubation attempts early.
- Avoid hypoxia.
- Ensure the failed intubation drill is clearly understood.

However, this is often unreliable and it is sensible to get another anaesthetist to be present for assistance if any difficulty is anticipated.

Use a standard laryngoscope first; this is what is familiar to all of us. Long-bladed laryngoscopes in small women often make for a difficult laryngoscopic view. Most delivery suites do not have a fibreoptic laryngoscope, but there is normally one in the main theatre block that can be transferred if needed. Pregnant women have a high metabolic rate and desaturate frighteningly quickly. Intubation needs to be performed swiftly and calmly.

Failed intubation drill

Failed intubation drill should be practised. The decision regarding what to do should have been thought out prior to the start of the anaesthetic. The important aspects of the drill are discussed in Box 8.2, and a sample failed intubation drill is shown in Box 8.3.

Repeated attempts at intubation are rarely successful. Turning the patient to the left lateral position takes time, and most anaesthetists are better at maintaining ventilation with the patient supine. A laryngeal mask may provide a patent airway but has the disadvantage of failing to protect the lungs from aspiration. This, however, is of secondary importance, as oxygenation is the priority. The decision as to whether to awaken the patient depends on the severity of the maternal and fetal condition. General anaesthesia must be continued if the mother's life depends upon surgery being completed. This is rare, and occurs in cases of maternal cardiac arrest, major haemorrhage or severe placental abruption. The anaesthetist has a primary responsibility to ensure that the mother is not harmed, but the decision between the fetus and the mother is not always easy to make. If ventilation is easy using an airway or a laryngeal mask, then consideration should be given to using a competitive relaxant and ventilating the patient. A 'heaving', spontaneously breathing patient is prone to regurgitation and vomiting; this also makes surgery more difficult.

Aspiration

Aspiration still occurs, and can be silent or obvious to the anaesthetist. Patients at high risk are those having an emergency

---

Box 8.2. Considerations for an obstetric failed intubation drill

- Call for help early.
- Maintain oxygenation.
- Consider whether a change of equipment or head position will improve the chances of intubation.
- Does removing cricoid pressure improve the view?
- Make an early decision as to whether intubation is possible.
- Have a low threshold for awakening the patient – is awake intubation possible?
- Do not give a second dose of relaxant to prolong intubation attempts.
- Leave patient in the supine, left lateral tilt position – it is easier to ventilate like this than in full lateral position.
- Convert to regional anaesthesia if at all possible.
- If general anaesthesia is to continue, consider using a laryngeal mask and assisted ventilation rather than spontaneous ventilation.
- Consider a Combitube (tracheal/oesophageal tube).
- Only use cricothyroidotomy as a last resort when the patient is unable to be ventilated.

Box 8.3. Failed intubation drill

- If you are unable to intubate, call for help; reposition the head and neck. Make a second attempt, and if successful, proceed. If the second attempt fails, ventilate with 100 per cent oxygen via facemask and airway. Consider LMA.
- If able to ventilate: if the airway is good and the patient is easy to ventilate, consider whether the procedure needs to continue, or if the patient can be woken up for a regional technique.
- If unable to ventilate: if the patient is not hypoxic, maintain an airway as best you can and wake the patient up. If the patient is hypoxic, consider airway manoeuvres as in Box 8.2 – ease cricoid pressure, use Combitube, cricothyroidotomy.

Caesarean section who have been given pethidine in labour without prophylactic antacid therapy. Aspiration pneumonitis is said to occur if greater than 25 ml of gastric content of pH > 3.5 enters the lung parenchyma. There is little evidence to substantiate this claim. Prevention by correct anaesthetic technique is the best solution, and a high index of suspicion should exist, especially in a patient who develops wheeze and low oxygen saturation. Treatment is supportive and may involve intensive care. The decision as to whether such a patient should be extubated at the end of the case is difficult to assess other than on an individual basis, but if the condition is not severe it is often prudent to extubate, and observe the mother. Mendelson's syndrome is named after Curtis L. Mendelson, who was a New York obstetrician. He first described this condition to the New York Obstetrical Society on 11 December 1941, and published his findings in the American Journal of Obstetrics and Gynecology in 1946 (vol. 52, pp. 191–204). Of 66 cases that involved aspiration only three died, and these were from tracheal obstruction by 'solid' vomit. He made several worthwhile points, some of which are still being reinforced today. These include the withholding of food in labour, the wider use of local anaesthetic techniques, alkalinization and emptying of the stomach contents, competent anaesthetic technique, and adequate anaesthetic equipment.

Postoperative analgesia

Caesarean section under general anaesthesia is painful. Up to 20 mg of intravenous morphine may be needed intraoperatively to provide a comfortable patient in the immediate postoperative phase. It is usual thereafter to prescribe either intramuscular or intravenous opiates (via a PCA pump) and, if not contraindicated, a regular non-steroidal analgesic either orally or via the rectal route.

9

The third stage of labour

The third stage of labour includes the early postpartum period from the birth of the infant to the delivery of the afterbirth (cord, placenta and membranes). It is usually uneventful, but it is a period of potential high maternal risk. Attention is usually focused on the neonate, and bleeding from genital tract trauma, episiotomy wounds or the uterus may be copious and unobserved. Thus as an anaesthetist called to provide postnatal anaesthesia, it is vital to assess the cardiovascular status of the patient carefully (pulse, blood pressure, capillary refill time and peripheral temperature are all valuable indicators) and try to estimate blood loss. If any doubt exists as to the degree of loss, or if the loss is prolonged, full resuscitation must be undertaken as part of anaesthetic intervention. Blood crossmatch should be considered early.

Active management of a normal third stage
Active management of the third stage (as opposed to a 'natural' third stage) is the use of an oxytocic agent, cord clamping and controlled cord traction to deliver the placenta. The prophylactic use of an oxytocic such as oxytocin 5–10 iu intravenously or syntometrine (500 μg ergometrine and 5 iu oxytocin) intramuscularly reduces the risk of major postpartum haemorrhage by up to 40 per cent.

Genital tract trauma
Perineal lacerations are common after childbirth, especially in centres where episiotomy is commonly used. Most are minor and can be sutured under local anaesthesia, perineal blockade, spinal analgesia or an epidural top-up. If bleeding is severe (classically seen with cervical tears) or the tear extends into the rectum or pelvis, regional or general anaesthesia is always required. As stated above, the preoperative assessment must be careful to exclude or treat hypovolaemia. Suggested block doses are listed in Box 9.1.

Box 9.1. Regimens for third stage anaesthesia

- Saddle block. This is suitable for first- or second-degree tears and repair of vaginal or cervical lacerations. The dose should be given with the patient in the sitting position, and she should be kept sitting up for at least 3–4 minutes, to ensure good sacral analgesia. Third-degree tears need full epidural blockade, and may require general anaesthesia if laparotomy or colostomy is performed. Epidural top-up: bupivacaine 0.5% 10 ml. Spinal: heavy bupivacaine 0.5% 1–1.5 ml.
- Evacuation of retained placenta. This can be an unpleasant procedure that requires full uterine and perineal anaesthesia, so a block similar to that for instrumental delivery is required (S_3–T_{10}). Epidural top-up: bupivacaine 0.5% 15–20 ml plus fentanyl 25–50 μg. Spinal: heavy bupivacaine 0.5% 2.0–2.5 ml.

Specific problems in the third stage

Uterine atony

The failure of the uterus to contract rapidly after delivery may be idiopathic, but several precipitating causes must be excluded. The commonest problem is a fully or partially retained placenta. This not only bleeds copiously of its own right, but also prevents contraction of the vessel-rich upper segment of the uterus, leading to further loss from the uterine decidua. Manual evacuation is used in preference to an instrumental procedure as the cervix is still widely dilated (this permits passage of the obstetrician's arm) and the ability to 'feel' the cavity decreases the risk of perforation. Once it is established that the cavity is clear, an infusion of oxytocin at 10 iu/h is often sufficient to ensure contraction. Rubbing the uterus vigorously through the anterior abdominal wall (or directly at laparotomy or during Caesarean section) also encourages contraction. Prostaglandins such as carbiprost (Hemabate®) can be used in refractory cases although contraindicated in asthmatics, and ergometrine is still regarded as effective although it is less popular due to its adverse side-effect profile (nausea, vomiting, and severe, prolonged vasoconstriction leading to hypertension).

Sepsis can also lead to uterine atony, and mothers with prolonged rupture of membranes should all be given antibiotic cover (as β-haemolytic streptococci are the commonest causative organisms, co-amoxiclav 8-hourly 375 mg orally or 1.2 g intravenously is appropriate). In these cases the bleeding may be torrential, and early consultant involvement, activation of the major haemorrhage protocol, invasive monitoring to guide aggressive resuscitation, and ITU involvement are to be advised.

Placenta accreta, increta and percreta

Occasionally the placenta is abnormally attached to the uterine wall. If the placenta invades through the decidua it is described as accreta; through the inner muscle layer as increta; and right through the uterine wall into the pelvis as percreta. Overall, maternal mortality from invasive placenta is quoted at 3 per cent, but this rises to 20 per cent in placenta percreta involving the bladder. Modern scanning ensures that the majority of these cases are detected antenatally so that appropriate precautions can be taken (eight-plus units of blood cross-matched, senior staff present, surgical removal of the placenta with prior consent for hysterectomy if required). It may be that the first presentation is of a partially retained placenta, and in these cases activation of a major haemorrhage alert and summoning senior support are immediate steps.

These cases can lead to massive haemorrhage, not only from placental vessels in the ingrown area but also from the disrupted uterine tissue failing to contract properly. This is initially managed as uterine atony, but if pharmacological methods fail to produce contraction and vasoconstriction it is necessary to consider early laparotomy for direct compression, packing, or hysterectomy.

Inverted uterus

Delivery of the placenta via cord traction can cause the uterus to invert. This is intensely painful and produces profound shock out of proportion to the blood loss. Intravenous glyceryl trinitrate (GTN) can be administered as 100–200 µg bolus doses to relax the cervix enough to push the fundus back. If this is not successful, general anaesthesia using a high-dose volatile agent (classically halothane, but isoflurane is effective) is required to relax the uterus. The shock reverses quickly once the inversion is corrected.

Epidural analgesia may be insufficient in these cases for three reasons. Hypotension may occur as a result of the inversion, rendering regional anaesthesia inappropriate. The block required for vaginal delivery is often not high enough to cover the visceral pain associated with an inversion, and there is no direct uterine relaxant effect on the muscle tissue. Administration of any procontractant drugs should obviously be avoided or ceased until the inversion is reversed.

10

Haemorrhage and other emergencies

Haemorrhage

Normal delivery is associated with a blood loss of less than 500 ml, and a blood loss of greater than 1000 ml is generally defined as a major haemorrhage. Its severity depends on the speed and volume of loss as well as the cause of the haemorrhage.

Major obstetric haemorrhage can kill, and is a leading cause of maternal mortality. The reported incidence varies from about 1 : 600–1 : 1000 deliveries. It may be visible (abrupt or a continuous ongoing ooze) or concealed, and may occur antepartum, at delivery or in the postpartum period.

Haemorrhage can occur from the uterus (atony, placenta praevia/accreta/retained placenta/abruption), from genital tract trauma (cervix, vaginal wall) or as a result of a coagulopathy. Patients who are particularly susceptible are those with placenta praevia on a previous uterine scar, and the control of haemorrhage in this group may necessitate a Caesarean hysterectomy.

It is important to realize that the normal clinical signs of late pregnancy can be similar to the early signs of ongoing haemorrhage. These include tachycardia and hyperventilation with a dilutional anaemia. The more obvious cardiovascular signs of haemorrhage such as hypotension may not develop until the blood volume is reduced by as much as 35 per cent, at a level of about 2 l blood loss. Pregnant patients are young and therefore have a good ability to compensate physiologically for hypotension. The uteroplacental circulation is at risk in haemorrhage due to compensatory vasoconstriction and diversion of the blood away from the uterine circulation to the more critical organs. This is worsened by the lack of an autoregulatory capacity in the placental circulation. Uterine blood flow is primarily determined by maternal blood pressure.

Failure to appreciate the amount of loss, especially in an ongoing 'ooze' situation, is one of the clinical difficulties encountered.

A high index of suspicion for haemorrhage should exist in the mind of the anaesthetist. Hypotension after regional anaesthesia is not always caused by the anaesthetist!

Management

Management revolves around early correct diagnosis, adequate resuscitation, and good communication with the obstetricians, blood transfusion/haematology service, porters and midwives. Ideally the blood transfusion/haematology service should be on the same site as the maternity unit. All maternity units are recommended to have protocols or guidelines regarding haemorrhage and to practise 'drills' regarding the management of massive haemorrhage. Most units carry two units of uncross-matched O-negative blood in the blood refrigerator. A suitable policy is shown in Box 10.1.

The basis of treatment is to treat the underlying cause, and often surgery is required, with ligation of the internal iliac arteries and hysterectomy being necessary in some cases. Radiological intervention with embolization of the bleeding arteries can prove curative. Disseminated intravascular coagulation is a secondary phenomenon that rapidly develops in these patients. It is rapidly triggered by depletion of clotting factors, by the release of procoagulant factors into the circulation, or by damage to the vascular endothelium. The delays in receiving coagulation profile results rapidly from laboratory services often means that it is obvious clinically before it is evident from laboratory results. Therefore, it is sensible to order fresh frozen plasma and platelets when ordering the blood.

Box 10.1. Guidelines for massive obstetric haemorrhage

- Notify haematology department – state obstetric haemorrhage, degree of urgency, cross-match 10 units of blood.
- Notify senior anaesthetists.
- Normovolaemia is the priority – give crystalloid or colloid 20 ml/kg intravenously.
- Monitor patient – urinary output, consider central venous access.
- Correct clotting abnormalities with platelets, cryoprecipitate, fresh frozen plasma.
- Notify HDU/ITU of patient.
- Treat cause – surgical? medical?
- Treat uterine dystonia (see Box 10.2).

Box 10.2. Uterine dystonia: treatment and major side effects

Treatment – Major side eects
Oxytocin 5–10 units as intravenous bolus, or by infusion – Hypotension, water intoxication, hyponatraemia
Ergometrine 0.25 mg diluted i.v. – Vomiting, hypertension and bronchospasm
Prostaglandin $F_{2\alpha}$ 0.25 mg i.m. or intramyometrial – Vomiting, hypertension, bronchospasm, intrapulmonary shunt
Prostaglandin E_2 5–20 μg/min i.v. – Both hypotension and hypertension reported

---

Anaesthesia for patients with haemorrhage can be difficult. The benefits versus the risks of regional anaesthesia when compared to general anaesthesia need to be carefully evaluated. In a patient who is normovolaemic with cardiovascular stability, regional blockade may be considered. Ongoing haemorrhage often necessitates general anaesthesia and transfer to HDU/ITU for ongoing care. Induction agents need to be given cautiously. Ketamine and etomidate cause minimal hypotension. Ketamine increases uterine tone and may assist if uterine atony exists, but also may aggravate fetal distress or abruptio placentae. Volatile agents generally relax the uterus at high doses, but it is known that isoflurane at a concentration of 0.5 MAC does not affect uterine tone.

Abruptio placentae

This is the premature separation of a normally implanted placenta from the uterus prior to the third stage of labour. Bleeding may be external (visible via the cervix) or concealed (within the uterine cavity). Assessment of blood loss is difficult in both cases and often inadequate. Coagulopathy is common in this condition. Fetal mortality is high, and is proportionate to the degree of placental separation. Maternal factors associated with abruption include increasing age and parity, hypertension, trauma, uterine abnormalities, premature rupture of membranes, and a previous history of abruption. It commonly presents as hypertonic uterine contractions, abdominal pain, vaginal bleeding, and/or severe fetal distress. Normovolaemia and the absence of a coagulopathy are necessary prior to considering regional anaesthesia. General anaesthesia is often needed, and these cases often constitute true emergencies in the delivery suite.

Placenta praevia

This is the implantation of the placenta over or near the uterine internal os. It is classified in the following manner:

- Grade 1 – a low-lying placenta praevia implanted in the lower uterine segment
- Grade 2 – a marginal placenta praevia lying proximate to the internal os
- Grade 3 – a partial placenta praevia in which the internal os is partially covered by placenta
- Grade 4 – a total or complete placenta praevia in which the internal os is totally covered by placenta.

The incidence is about 0.5 per cent of all deliveries. Maternal risk factors are increasing age, high parity, previous Caesarean section, and previous miscarriage. It manifests itself as painless haemorrhage normally after 30 weeks' gestation. If diagnosed in the second trimester a spontaneous resolution rate of 90 per cent occurs due to placental migration from lower segment growth in the last trimester. In cases of marginal or low-lying placenta praevia vaginal delivery may be considered, but the risk of haemorrhage is high. Caesarean section is often the delivery method of choice. Both regional and general anaesthesia are used, although there is debate about the choice of technique in grade 4 praevia. Regional anaesthesia in major haemorrhage can be difficult in that managing a hypotensive, bleeding, awake patient can be fraught. Conversion to general anaesthesia mid-surgery in this situation is also difficult, and for these reasons general anaesthesia is often preferred at the outset. Anaesthetists must be aware of the catastrophic bleeding that can occur, especially in those mothers with a previous uterine scar. Blood should be present in the theatre and it is sensible to have two large-bore intravenous lines established prior to surgery, and the cross-matched blood in the labour ward refrigerator.

Women presenting with placenta praevia and a previous uterine scar from a Caesarean section must be suspected of having placenta accreta, and have a greater tendency to haemorrhage; they may require Caesarean hysterectomy.

Ruptured uterus

Classically this occurs when vaginal delivery is considered a suitable method of delivery in a patient who has had a previous Caesarean section (trial of scar). Rupture, however, does occur in the un-scarred uterus, and is thought to be due to two major factors: grand parity and excessive oxytocin use. It presents with a sudden increase in abdominal pain experienced in the labouring woman, fetal distress, and vaginal bleeding. The pain of the rupture will be felt by the mother even when low-dose epidural analgesia is used, and it may present as inadequate pain relief after epidural analgesia. A high level of suspicion is needed for the diagnosis. Delivery of the fetus by Caesarean section is mandatory, and the anaesthetic tech-nique chosen depends on the degree of fetal distress present and the time available.

Amniotic fluid embolism

At term there is about 1 l of amniotic fluid present, but the volume necessary to enter the circulation and cause clinical effects is un-known. Amniotic fluid embolism is extremely rare and is said to occur classically in elderly multiparous mothers with large babies following a rapid labour associated with syntocinon use. It presents with respiratory distress, cyanosis, cardiovascular collapse, con-vulsions, haemorrhage, disseminated intravascular coagulation, convulsions or pulmonary oedema. A definitive diagnosis can only be made by finding amniotic fluid elements in the maternal circulation – certainly a post-event and often a postmortem diagnosis. Treatment requires intensive care therapy and is aimed at maternal cardiovascular support, volume replacement and treatment of any bleeding diatheses.

External cephalic version

Anaesthetists are often notified of this procedure for the manage-ment of breech presentation in late pregnancy. There is no anaes-thetic involvement with this planned procedure but the woman should be fasted prior to it, as fetal distress requiring Caesarean section is a real possibility. Fetal dysrhythmias are common in the procedure. Other reported complications include haemorrhage, abruption, membrane rupture and amniotic fluid embolism.

Cord prolapse

Cord prolapse is a rare but serious complication of multiple preg-nancies, or those in which the fetus is small, there is premature labour or a breech presentation. Cord compression must be avoided and the mother prepared for Caesarean section. Regional anaesthesia can be used successfully if there is no cord compression or fetal distress.

The dead fetus

Placental abruption and cord/fetal abnormalities account for the majority of late fetal deaths. Spontaneous labour normally begins about 2 weeks after intrauterine death, and for this reason labour is often induced. Coagulation disorders and thrombocytopenia can occur, although normally the fetus will have been dead for over 4 weeks in these cases. Necrotic fetal tissue causes the release of thromboplastin and coagulation cascade activation. Epidural analgesia can be used for analgesia and delivery if not contraindicated.

Sepsis

Puerperal sepsis continues to be a major source of maternal mortality; the genital tract in general and the uterine bed in particular are fertile sites for infective organisms. Common causal agents are haemolytic streptococci and *E. coli*. Antibiotic prophylaxis is mandatory for all operative procedures for this reason.

If puerperal sepsis is suspected, swabs and blood cultures should be taken prior to antibiotic dosing. HDU care should be considered early.

11

Pre-eclampsia and eclampsia

Pre-eclampsia is a disease characterized by raised blood pressure, proteinurea and peripheral oedema that occurs more commonly amongst young primiparous women. It presents as a spectrum of conditions ranging from a relatively benign hypertensive state that can be present for some months to convulsions in a previously asymptomatic woman. The complications are rare but can be fatal.

Definitions

The terms pre-eclampsia, gestational proteinuric hypertension and pregnancy-induced hypertension are all in common usage. The hypertension component has been defined by the International Society for the Study of Hypertension in Pregnancy as a single diastolic reading (phase V) of 110 mmHg or above, or two readings of 90 mmHg or greater at least 4 hours apart, occurring after the twentieth week of pregnancy in a previously normotensive woman. An American working group has defined it as a rise of greater than 15 mmHg diastolic or greater than 30 mmHg systolic compared with readings taken earlier in pregnancy. The latter definition allows for the identification of women with hypertension superimposed upon chronic hypertension. A diastolic blood pressure of greater than 90 mmHg before 20 weeks suggests chronic hypertension. Whether the phase IV or phase V component of blood pressure is measured is open to discussion. Many mechanical non-invasive blood pressure machines measure phase V, which produces a reading of about 5 mmHg less than phase IV.

The proteinuric component is defined as a protein concentration of greater than 0.3 g/l in a 24-hour urine collection. This is not routinely measured, and reliance is placed on urine Reagent Strip testing. A 2+ strip test on two occasions 4 hours apart is used, and equates with a 24-hour collection with a total protein of greater than 0.3 g/l.

Oedema is an unreliable indicator and is common in normal pregnancy. In pre-eclampsia it is usually more generalized and is not just confined to the ankles and sacral area.

Eclampsia is defined as a generalized convulsion occurring during pregnancy, labour, or within 7 days of delivery in the absence of epilepsy or any other disorder predisposing to convulsions. The severity of the disease is often assessed biochemically by measuring urate levels (with a level >450 mmol/l indicating severe pre-eclampsia), an indicator of renal tubular function.

Clinical features

The disease may affect all the organ systems listed in Box 11.1. Presentation is rare before 24 weeks' gestation (presentation at 20 weeks has been reported in association with hydatidiform mole), and often asymptomatic hypertension and proteinurea are discovered at a routine antenatal check-up. The presentation can be abrupt and severe at the other end of the spectrum, and it is not unknown for the first presentation to be eclampsia. Epigastric pain from liver distension is an important clinical sign. The HELLP syndrome is haemolysis, elevated liver enzymes (AST >50) and low platelets. Intracranial haemorrhage is still a major cause of mortality in these patients. Signs and symptoms resolve normally within 48 hours of delivery, but ITU/HDU management is mandatory, and early hepatology involvement wise.

Aetiology and pathology

Failure of spiral artery relaxation in the placenta is the primary problem in this disease. The cause is thought to be immunological,

---

Box 11.1. Systemic effects of pre-eclampsia

- Cardiovascular: intravascular hypovolaemia, elevated systemic vascular resistance, hyperdynamic left ventricular function.
- Placenta: abruptio placenta, intra-uterine growth retardation.
- Respiratory: pulmonary oedema.
- Renal: proteinurea, acute renal failure.
- Nervous system: headache, hyperreflexia, visual disturbances, eclampsia and cerebral haemorrhage.
- Hepatic: liver dysfunction, HELLP syndrome, periportal necrosis, subcapsular haematoma and epigastric pain.
- Haematological: thrombocytopenia, haemolysis and disseminated intravascular coagulation.

but the mechanism is unclear although it is perhaps from an increased response to fetal antigens. The conversion processes involved in this placental and immunological disorder becoming a multisystem disease are unknown. In the placenta there is a failure of trophoblastic invasion of the arterial walls and arterial blockade by macrophages, platelets and fibrin. Placental blood flow reduction occurs, with resulting placental ischaemia. This is followed by release of a humoral factor that causes widespread endothelial damage, and this leads to the multisystemic effects that result.

The hypertension was traditionally considered to be due to an elevated systemic vascular resistance with a low intravascular volume. However, it has now been shown that hyperdynamic left ventricular function is also causative. In the lungs, both a damaged pulmonary vascular endothelium and low colloid osmotic pressure account for the pulmonary oedema that can be seen at low central venous pressures. In pre-eclampsia both renal blood flow and glomerular filtration rate are decreased by about 30 per cent; however, this is still above normal non-pregnant levels. Changes in renal parenchyma are completely reversed after delivery. Rarely, acute tubular necrosis occurs, and again this is associated with full renal recovery if managed correctly.

Management

Management is coordinated with the obstetricians and the patient should ideally be managed in an obstetric high dependency area. A midwife trained in the management of medically ill patients should care for her on a one-to-one basis. Delivery is the ultimate cure of the disease. Management should focus upon the control of hypertension, appropriate fluid management, maintenance of renal perfusion and urine output, and the supportive management of complications. Monitoring of oxygen saturation and supplemental oxygen may be necessary.

Hypertension is managed by drug therapy. Methyldopa 250 mg–1 g three times a day is traditionally used orally pre-delivery as it is not teratogenic (larger doses cause maternal sedation). Oral (100 mg twice daily) or intravenous (5–10 mg bolus doses) labetalol is used in addition if required. The directly acting vasodilator hydralazine (5–10 mg intravenously over 10 minutes as a bolus or a maintenance infusion of 50–150 µg/min) is the current mainstay of labour ward management, but tachyphylaxis is a problem with continued use. Magnesium is effective due to its direct vasodilator effect. Oral or sublingual nifedipine (5–10 mg to three times a day) is also used. The blood pressure should be lower than the arbitrarily defined figures of 140/90, and should be recorded every 15 minutes in the acute situation. In severe cases a direct measurement device is helpful.

Fluid therapy is normally given as a maintenance dose of crystalloid (normal saline or Hartmann's solution at 2 l/day). Should urine output be inadequate (less than 0.5 ml/kg per hour) then central venous catheter insertion and pressure measurement should be considered. Excessive fluid therapy can precipitate pulmonary oedema but inadequate fluid causes renal impairment, so the insertion of a central venous catheter is sometimes indicated. Internal jugular vein cannulation can be difficult in oedematous patients, and there are reports of life-threatening airway obstruction occurring from accidental puncture of the carotid artery in these patients. These patients may have abnormal coagulation profiles as well, and for these reasons it is often sensible to insert an antecubital fossa long line.

Eclampsia is considered to be due to cerebral vasospasm. It is initially managed with the primary resuscitation therapy of airway control, left lateral positioning, oxygen therapy, termination of the convulsion, and urgent delivery of the fetus if indicated. Further convulsions should be prevented. Specific drug therapy to stop the convulsion includes any of: intravenous diazepam 5–10 mg (which is easily available in the delivery suite); intravenous thiopentone if in the operating theatre environment; or intravenous magnesium sulphate (Box 11.2) 4 g slowly over up to 5 minutes (this is a cerebral vasodilator).

Magnesium is indicated after eclampsia to prevent further convulsions for 24–48 hours. The clinical and side effects correlate fairly well with the plasma levels of magnesium (Box 11.3).

Toxicity can be assessed clinically by measuring the tendon reflexes. If absent, the drug infusion regimen should be reviewed and blood levels taken. Tendon reflexes in the lower limbs may be decreased or absent if epidural anaesthesia has been given.

Anaesthesia for the pre-eclamptic patient
Regional anaesthesia
Regional anaesthesia can be used without problems in the majority of asymptomatic mild pre-eclamptic patients. Coagulation and platelet profiles should be known before commencing regional anaesthetic techniques, and a platelet count of greater than

---

Box 11.2. Use of magnesium sulphate in eclampsia

- Presentation: as 50% magnesium sulphate, 10 ml ampoules containing 5 g (20 mmol).
- Dose: intravenous bolus followed by infusion, 4 g (40–80 mg/kg) over a minimum of 5 minutes followed by a maintenance infusion of 1–2 g/h.
- Side effects: drowsiness, sedation, headache, blurred vision, nausea, constipation, hypotension, cardiac arrhythmias, pulmonary oedema, loss of reflexes, prolongation of neuromuscular blockade.
- Overdose management: stop drug, supportive treatment, assess blood levels, and consider 10 ml slow intravenous calcium gluconate or chloride 10%.
- Recurrent seizures: additional bolus 2 g magnesium over 5 minutes with 2 g repeated if necessary 15 minutes later.

Box 11.3. Magnesium: clinical effects and plasma levels

	Plasma levels (mmol/l)
Normal levels	0.7–1.0
Therapeutic levels	2.0–3.5
Widened QRS complex and prolonged PR interval	>3.0
Sedation, severe headache, blurred vision	>4.0
Absent tendon reflexes	>5.0
Heart block, respiratory paralysis, cardiac arrest	7.5–14.0

80×10^9/l is acceptable. Caution should be exercised in patients who have an ongoing downward spiral of platelet numbers, as this is an indication of disease severity. Risks must be compared to benefits. A decision must be taken by the anaesthetist as to whether spinal or epidural anaesthesia is used for operative procedures. The problems of regional anaesthesia are that spinal anaesthesia, with the rapid onset sympathetic blockade that is produced, can lead to profound hypotension. Intravenous administration of large volumes of fluid and use of ephedrine can precipitate pulmonary oedema and heart failure in the acutely ill patient. This is more marked in patients who are not on antihypertensive drug therapy. Many people advocate spinal anaesthesia despite this problem but, time permitting, a carefully incrementally topped-up epidural catheter in the severely ill patient leads to less fluid therapy being given, less cardiovascular strain and a more stable clinical situation. An epidural catheter can also be used to manage any postoperative analgesia.

General anaesthesia

General anaesthesia is also potentially hazardous, and is normally undertaken only if regional anaesthesia is contraindicated. Three specific problems arise in this situation: the patient may have cardiac failure and pulmonary oedema; intubation may be difficult due to airway oedema; and intubation and extubation may exaggerate hypertensive pressor responses. Existing antihypertensive medication should be continued if possible. Untreated patients may be given incremental labetalol or hydralazine to reduce the blood pressure pre-induction. The hypertensive response can be attenuated by the intravenous administration of alfentanil 10–20 µg/kg. The paediatrician must be informed of the fact that the baby may be sedated. Esmolol can cause fetal bradycardia and is not recommended as a suitable agent in this situation although, in a dose of 1 mg/kg, it may be of benefit in avoiding extubation pressor responses.

Postoperatively, prudence must be exercised when prescribing non-steroidal anti-inflammatory drugs to patients with severe preeclampsia, as any renal damage might be aggravated and platelet function may be impaired.

12

Intercurrent disease, pregnancy and labour

It is often assumed that the mortality and morbidity associated with pregnancy and childbirth is related purely to the physiological and pathophysiological changes associated with these events. Whilst this is true in the main, there is an increasingly large cohort of women with potentially severe systemic disease who wish to have children. These include patients with relatively early onset of adult systemic disorders (hypertension, coronary artery disease) and those who have survived childhood or congenital disease with lasting sequelae (corrected congenital heart lesions, cystic fibrosis, motor neurone disease). This group also includes mothers whose systemic disease is revealed by the increased physiological stress of pregnancy (e.g. mitral valve disease, glomerulonephritis) and those who have impaired control of their disease as a result of pregnancy (e.g. insulin dependent diabetics, multiple sclerosis sufferers who have stopped interferon). These patients present a challenge both to the obstetrician and the anaesthetist, and early liaison between those managing the pregnancy and the relevant specialities is vital.

Cardiovascular disease

In the UK 0.3–5 per cent of parturients have definable cardiac disease, and the incidence of adults with congenital disease is rising as survival to maturity increases. The valvular lesions associated with rheumatic fever are less commonly seen. The exception to this is in the immigrant community, where significant rheumatic mitral valve stenosis is often missed until it presents acutely as atrial fibrillation with heart failure. Also, the increasingly ageing obstetric population has higher risk of acquired cardiac disease due to smoking, hypertension, diabetes and diet.

Against this background it is reassuring that the number of maternal deaths from cardiac disease has not increased over the last 20 years, despite the increase in 'at risk' patients. The most recent triennial report into maternal mortality suggests that this increase in high cardiac risk mothers is not only due to the improved survival into adulthood of those with congenital lesions. Attitude changes amongst high-risk mothers and the cardiologists and obstetricians who care for them mean that the right to have a baby is much more forcibly expressed and more likely to be assisted.

Reports indicate that major complicating features in cardiac obstetric fatalities are pulmonary hypertension and a past history of myocardial infarction or endocarditis. All patients presenting in pregnancy with cardiac symptoms or history should be assessed early and by cardiologists. As well as normal cardiorespiratory data, further investigations should be considered (see Box 12.1). These tests often need to be repeated throughout pregnancy, as increasing cardiac strain may lead to gradual decompensation. Antibiotic prophylaxis must be remembered in all mothers with structural or valvular lesions.

Labour and cardiac disease

Analgesic technique is determined by the disease severity, mode of delivery and anticoagulation status. Epidural analgesia will reduce catecholamine release but may require fluid loading and vasopressor therapy. In those with severe restrictive cardiac deficit regional anaesthesia may be impossible because of concerns about vasodilation leading to cardiovascular collapse due to fixed cardiac output, and these patients should not be allowed to labour.

Monitoring

Continuous ECG and blood pressure monitoring is essential, and central venous and arterial lines provide valuable information. The use of pulmonary artery catheters is controversial, and should be restricted to those with a New York Heart Association grade IV classification after discussion with cardiology and anaesthetic consultants.

- *Aortic stenosis* leads to a fixed cardiac output due to a reduced cross-sectional area in the outflow tract of the left ventricle. In asymptomatic patients vaginal delivery is often possible with careful monitoring, providing a low threshold for intervention is maintained. Symptomatic aortic stenosis is associated with left ventricular hypertrophy, ischaemia and conduction deficits (left bundle branch block in congenital cases), and increases

---

Box 12.1. Assessment of the 'cardiac risk' obstetric patient

Ideally, assessment begins prior to conception.

- Clinical assessment: exercise tolerance and shortness of breath, ankle swelling, angina, orthopnoea and paroxysmal nocturnal dyspnoea all need to be specifically asked about. Heart rate and rhythm, blood pressure and oxygen saturation should be measured and chest and cardiac auscultation performed; respiratory function testing may be considered if appropriate.
- Blood tests: haemoglobin, renal function. Arterial blood gas analysis may be considered.
- Radiology: a chest radiograph used to be indicated to assess the cardiac shadow and lung fields, but this has been replaced by dynamic ultrasonographic and Doppler imaging.
- Electrocardiographic tests: a 12-lead ECG is mandatory; 24-hour Holter monitoring (for arrhythmias) or exercise testing (for ischaemic change) may also be indicated.
- Echocardiography: recently data tables for normal values in middle and late pregnancies have been published, and these enable both quantitative and qualitative changes to be assessed non-invasively. Transoesophageal echocardiography provides better images, but may require maternal sedation. It is a useful tool in the perioperative or ITU management of high-risk patients.
- Invasive imaging and intervention: cardiac catheterization ± angioplasty or stenting may be a life-saving procedure in the acutely decompensated or infarcting mother.

---

mortality and morbidity risk for both mother and baby. A prolonged PR interval on ECG suggests a high risk of complete heart block developing. Management is to ensure that normal heart rate and blood pressure is maintained as well as a normal venous return. Inotropic therapy is often indicated, and in severe cases a cardiac anaesthetic technique (high opioid – fentanyl 20 µg/kg; low volatile to decrease vasodilation) may be needed for Caesarean section under general anaesthesia. In all cases the neonatal unit must be warned, as the fetus may need ventilation and runs a greater than normal risk of hypoxia secondary to placental hypoperfusion.

- *Mitral stenosis* is rarely seen in First World parturients. It is associated with immigrants from areas where rheumatic fever is still common. Avoidance of tachycardia facilitates left atrial emptying and thus lowers left atrial pressure, and increases stroke volume. Atrial fibrillation is best treated with digoxin or, in the case of acute decompensation, cardioversion.

- *Pulmonary hypertension* is usually seen in pregnancy as a primary disease rather than secondary to chronic respiratory disease. Maintenance of venous return and avoidance of hypoxia and acidosis are vital to prevent rises in pulmonary vascular resistance and subsequent right ventricular failure. A prostacyclin infusion can be used centrally to decrease vascular resistance, but this may also have systemic effects and should be used with extreme care. Oxytocin may aggravate this.
- *Cardiac arrhythmias* are more common during pregnancy, especially supraventricular tachycardias. If the maternal condition is compromised or fetoplacental perfusion falls, electrical cardioversion is relatively safe and effective. Patients fitted with pacemakers or implanted defibrillators should be assessed prior to becoming pregnant if possible, or as soon as their cardiology team knows of the pregnancy.
- *Congenital heart lesions* and intracardiac shunts represent an area of particularly high maternal risk. Cyanotic (right-to-left) shunts in particular are associated with high maternal mortality. Atrial shunts tend not to be problematic unless associated with pulmonary artery stenosis. Interventricular and aortopulmonary shunts represent a much more serious management problem. Maternal Eisenmenger syndrome (pulmonary hypertension, right-to-left or bi-directional shunting and cyanosis) is associated with 30 per cent maternal mortality after spontaneous delivery and 50 per cent after Caesarean section. Falls in systemic vascular resistance must be aggressively treated with vasopressor agents to prevent an increase in right-to-left shunt, and high-flow oxygen therapy maintained to prevent hypoxic pulmonary vasoconstriction. Pre-existing polycythaemia worsens after delivery, and there is an associated increased risk of pulmonary embolism.
- *Ischaemic heart disease* associated with smoking, hypertension, diabetes, obesity and hypercholesterolaemia is increasingly common. Medical optimization and full collaboration with cardiologists is vital. Pre-delivery angiography and angioplasty may be necessary.
- *Hypertrophic cardiomyopathy* tends to be problematic only if myocardial work is significantly increased by increased vascular resistance or venous return. Gradual establishment of epidural blockade is often beneficial for these reasons.
- *Coarctation of the aorta* is usually corrected in early childhood, but for those with uncorrected lesions blood pressure control

should be maintained rigorously throughout pregnancy and labour as there is a risk of aortic dissection if hypertension occurs.

Respiratory disease

Acute exacerbation of chronic respiratory disease is common in pregnancy and labour. Asthma is common in women of childbearing age, and other chronic disease states are also encountered (e.g. cystic fibrosis, tuberculosis, bronchiectasis). In addition, the first generation of premature infants with chronic obstructive pulmonary disease from prolonged neonatal ventilation are themselves having children. The challenge presented by these patients is often made worse by suboptimal maintenance therapy, and a respiratory specialist should review all patients in this category when they are known to be pregnant.

Acute respiratory problems are less common and may be due to many causes (see Box 12.2).

- *Chest infections* and *pneumonia* should be aggressively treated with antibiotics and physiotherapy, and oxygen therapy started much earlier than in the non-gravid woman. Maternal oxygen saturation must be maintained at over 94 per cent. This is because the fetus exists on the steep part of the oxygen dissociation curve, and any maternal drop in PaO_2 below about 8 kPa leads to a precipitous drop in fetal oxygenation.
- *Acute respiratory distress syndrome* (ARDS) is increasingly associated with maternal deaths in the triennial mortality reports. This probably represents improved initial resuscitation and ITU management for critically ill mothers – they are dying of late complications rather than initial ones.
- *Asthma* usually improves during pregnancy. This may in part be due to a reduction in smoking and stress but is also related to an improvement in bronchial responsiveness, which starts in the second trimester and is not associated with changes in plasma, cortisol or progesterone levels. All usual medication should be continued. Theophyllines are best avoided, as blood levels can vary widely and they can cause fetal irritability. Prostaglandins must not be used to induce labour, and non-steroidal analgesics must be avoided. A labouring woman who requires systemic steroids for her asthma, either acutely or chronically, should be given these intravenously. Acute asthma is managed in the same

---

Box 12.2. Causes of acute respiratory failure in pregnancy

General – intrapulmonary:

- ARDS.
- Aspiration of gastric contents.
- Pneumothorax.
- Anaphylaxis.
- Asthma.
- Pulmonary embolism.

General – non-pulmonary:

- Airway obstruction.
- Neuromuscular (muscular dystrophy, trauma, myasthenia).
- Neurological (intracranial pathology, opioids).

Pregnancy-specific:

- Amniotic fluid embolism.

---

way as in the non-pregnant patient. Full monitoring and blood gas analyses are vital, and in the event of deterioration early transfer to a high dependency area is advisable.

- *Cystic fibrosis* is an autosomal recessive disease of the exocrine glands leading to chronic inflammation, bronchiectasis and fibrosis. Repeated chest infections and chronic inflammation lead to progressively worsening lung damage. Despite cyclical penicillin and cephalosporin therapy throughout pregnancy, 30 per cent of pregnant women with cystic fibrosis will be admitted during pregnancy. Those with severe disease characteristically have an FEV_1 less than 60 per cent of predicted. These patients are likely to have cor pulmonale, severe airflow obstruction and hypoxaemia. They tend to deliver very prematurely, and suffer severe worsening of their condition during and after pregnancy. Those who have undergone heart–lung transplants may have the physiological reserve to survive pregnancy and labour, but the increased risks of rejection and major fetal malformation make pregnancy inadvisable. Treatment is multidisciplinary throughout pregnancy and labour, with physiotherapists and nutritionists playing a vital role. Epidural analgesia must be carefully monitored to prevent respiratory embarrassment. General anaesthesia should be avoided where possible, and humidification of gases used at all times.

Renal disease

Renal impairment or failure can occur in pregnancy de novo or as a worsening of a chronic state. Pregnancy-related pathology is the commonest cause of acute renal failure in young women (see Box 12.3), and this is usually part of a multisystem complication.

- Chronic renal disease is associated with a decrease in fertility. The chance of pregnancy precipitating a worsening of renal function is related to the initial severity of the disease. For those with *mild to moderate renal impairment* (plasma creatinine 120–250 µmol/l), pregnancy usually has little or no effect. Serious deterioration in function has been reported, particularly in those with lupus-related nephropathy (glomerular sclerosis). These patients are also more susceptible to uncontrolled hypertensive episodes, and infants are likely to be prematurely delivered and underweight for dates.
- In those with more *severe renal disease*, a fetal mortality rate of >50 per cent is expected and the effect on the remaining tubular function of the mother is often severe. Conception is often impossible without fertility augmentation. Women on *dialysis* usually need the interval between sessions to be shortened to remove the increased metabolic waste load and to prevent hypervolaemia. The anaemia associated with chronic renal failure is worsened in pregnancy, and repeated transfusions may be needed.
- Over 50 per cent of women who have a successful *renal transplant* have pre-term labour following spontaneous rupture of the membranes. One in ten will have a graft failure as a direct result of the pregnancy, and complications, including hypertension, cerebrovascular accidents and miscarriage, are more common in this population. Caesarean section may be complicated by the

---

Box 12.3. Causes of acute renal failure in pregnancy

- Direct nephrotoxicity – drugs (non-steroidal analgesics, antibiotics).
- Multisystem disease – pre-eclampsia, HELLP syndrome, immune complex disease.
- Shock – septic (chorioamnionitis, incomplete or septic abortion/termination), hypovolaemic (antepartum/postpartum haemorrhage), anaphylactoid (transfusion or drug reaction).

presence of the graft in the pelvis, rendering the procedure technically more difficult.

All pregnant women with renal disease should undergo serial measurement of plasma and urinary electrolytes, protein, urea and creatinine throughout pregnancy. Creatinine clearance should be regularly assessed and any evidence of deterioration treated promptly. Hypertension must also be aggressively treated in consultation with nephrologists.

In labour, epidural analgesia can be used with care. Fluid filling should be guided by central pressure monitoring if renal impairment is severe, and invasive monitoring in a high dependency area considered early if renal or obstetric complications occur. Potentially problematic commonly used drugs are listed in Box 12.4.

Hepatobiliary disease

The majority of liver disorders encountered in pregnancy arise as a result of the pregnancy itself (hyperemesis gravidarum, intrahepatic cholestasis of pregnancy), and may be related to pre-eclampsia (HELLP syndrome, acute fatty liver of pregnancy). Jaundice in pregnancy is rare, and always warrants investigation. The commonest cause is viral hepatitis, but intrahepatic cholestasis, gallstone disease, drug toxicity and alcoholic cirrhosis all need to be considered. Rarer causes include Budd–Chiari syndrome, primary biliary cirrhosis and cholangitis. Ultrasound is a useful diagnostic tool, but early review by hepatologists is vital. Liver biopsy is often indicated to ascertain the diagnosis.

- The commonest cause of elevated liver transaminases in pregnancy is *hyperemesis gravidarum*. Its cause is unclear, but it is associated with obesity, nulliparous mothers and multiple pregnancy, and occurs in approximately 0.5 per cent of pregnancies. Sufferers may require hospital admission for rehydration and symptom control.
- *Intrahepatic cholestasis of pregnancy* usually presents in the third trimester as severe pruritus followed later by obstructive jaundice. Maternal morbidity is severe but not dangerous (insomnia, anorexia and abdominal discomfort), and resolves spontaneously after delivery. Fetal mortality is increased up to five-fold from normal in some series, and early section should be considered if serial enzyme monitoring indicates that the mother's condition is deteriorating.

Box 12.4. Obstetric and anaesthetic drugs: problems in renal disease

---

- Volatile anaesthetics: isoflurane or sevoflurane are the agents of choice as they are almost exclusively exhaled unchanged. All volatile agents decrease glomerular filtration and renal blood flow.
- Muscle relaxants: avoid gallamine (it is of historical and multiple choice relevance only; it crosses the placenta), and ensure plasma potassium is normal prior to using suxamethonium. In severe disease atracurium is the relaxant of choice, as its offset is independent of renal function.
- Analgesics: non-steroidal anti-inflammatory drugs are contraindicated in all patients with renal impairment. Pethidine and tramadol have metabolites that are predominantly renally excreted and can cause prolonged toxic effects.
- Obstetric drugs: ergometrine is contraindicated in renal failure. Magnesium dosage should be reduced and levels monitored closely.

Neurological and neuromuscular disease

The spectrum of neurological disease is vast and complex. However, most patients presenting with a pregnancy and a known neurological condition should present a manageable challenge to the anaesthetist provided care is taken.

- *Epilepsy* is the commonest cause of convulsions during pregnancy, and seizure frequency increases mainly due to subtherapeutic levels of maintenance anticonvulsant therapy caused by altered pharmacokinetics and poor compliance. Anti-epileptic drugs may have teratogenic effects on the fetus, so careful preconception advice and follow-up during pregnancy is required from the neurologist. Other causes of seizure should always be remembered (Box 12.5). Continuous fetal and maternal monitoring and maternal supplemental oxygen are mandatory, and Caesarean section under general anaesthesia should be considered if any signs of fetal distress occur. In this case thiopentone is the ideal induction agent due to its profound anticonvulsant effect.
- *Cerebrovascular disease* occasionally presents catastrophically during labour as a maternal seizure followed by collapse and coma or cardiorespiratory arrest. In these cases rapid Caesarean section as part of cardiopulmonary resuscitation (see Chapter 14) ensures the best chance of a live fetus. Delivery more than 15

Box 12.5. Causes of convulsions during labour

- Hypoxia.
- Hypotension.
- Epilepsy.
- Eclampsia.
- Space-occupying intracranial lesion (abscess, tumour).
- Cerebrovascular event (intracerebral, subdural or extradural haemorrhage; sinus thrombosis).
- Drug effects (narcotic overdose or withdrawal; allergy; local anaesthetic toxicity).
- Metabolic derangement.
- Sepsis.
- Amniotic fluid embolus.

---

minutes post-arrest is associated with extremely poor fetal outcome.

- In mothers with a known lesion, such as a *central nervous system aneurysm* or *arteriovenous malformation*, the management of delivery is dependent on previous treatment. A clipped or repaired lesion should present no further hazard to the mother, who can be allowed to labour normally. Epidural analgesia is positively indicated both to prevent the hypertensive responses to contraction pain and to prevent the urge to push at full dilation. Instrumental delivery avoids the rises in intracranial pressure associated with pushing, and obstetric efforts should be timed to match the contractions. In women with an untreated lesion, delivery is usually a combined procedure under general anaesthesia, with craniotomy following the delivery. This obviously is an elective process that requires coordination between anaesthetist, obstetrician, neurosurgeon, paediatrician, theatres, and the adult and neonatal intensive care units. Invasive monitoring is vital, and extreme care must be taken to obtund any hypertensive response to intubation or surgery.
- Mothers with *intracranial shunts* may be managed in a similar way to those with clipped aneurysms. Prophylaxis with antibiotics is important, particularly if the shunt is peritoneal. Patients should be carefully observed for evidence of rising intracranial pressure. Shunt blockage is more common during pregnancy and labour, and needs urgent treatment if it occurs.

Peripheral neurological and neuromuscular disease presents a variety of problems. It used to be advised that regional anaesthetic techniques be avoided in these patients for medicolegal reasons (any worsening of the symptoms is 'blamed' on the epidural). This is no longer regarded as acceptable and, provided careful prenatal discussion and documentation of deficit is carried out, epidural analgesia is usually helpful.

- Patients with *paraplegia* and other *chronic spinal cord injuries* may have multisystem disease, and antenatal assessment by a senior obstetrician and anaesthetist is important. Autonomic hyper-reflexia is the main complication seen, when uterine contractions precipitate sympathetic outflow distal to the lesion, resulting in hypertension, headache and bradycardia in response to the intense vasoconstriction. Epidural anaesthesia prevents this and is important even in those who have a thoracic cord lesion (and therefore painless contractions).
- Epidural analgesia is also possible in those who have had *previous spinal surgery* or *laminectomy*. Patients should be warned that there is an increased risk of patchy block, failure and inadvertent dural puncture. Spinal anaesthesia is the technique of choice for Caesarean section, due to the increased risk of dural puncture with a Tuohy needle.
- *Myasthenia gravis* is an autoimmune disease characterized by asymmetric muscle fatigue that spreads and worsens as the disease progresses. Patients are treated mainly with long-acting anticholinesterases (pyridostigmine) and steroids. They are usually extremely knowledgeable about both their disease and their own functional ability, and should be fully consulted throughout the pregnancy. Respiratory function is usually monitored with serial peak flow readings, and vaginal delivery with epidural analgesia and an assisted second stage is ideal. Sedation is best avoided because of respiratory compromise. Aminoglycosides and magnesium should not be used as they worsen symptoms, and if general anaesthesia is unavoidable it must be remembered that muscle relaxant effects are prolonged, and postoperative respiratory support may be necessary. A myasthenic crisis is characterized by increasing muscle weakness progressing to respiratory failure, and is treated with intravenous edrophonium. Cholinergic crisis is diagnosed when muscarinic effects predominate, and is caused by excessive drug therapy. Treatment is supportive.

- *Dystrophia myotonica* is an autosomal dominant disorder of sarcoplasmic calcium control resulting in delayed relaxation after muscle contraction. This affects uterine muscle, so labour is often prolonged and contractions ineffective. Caesarean section under regional anaesthesia is the preferred method, with aggressive warming of the patient to prevent shivering, as this provokes myotonic crisis. Suxamethonium is contraindicated as it caused masseter spasm, and patients are extremely sensitive to anaesthetic and analgesic drugs. Myotonic crisis/spasm does not relax with regional anaesthesia, and must be treated with quinine or dantrolene. High dependency care is advisable, and careful monitoring of respiratory function is vital.
- *Multiple sclerosis* presents no direct problem to the anaesthetist provided that prenatal assessment has indicated an adequate respiratory reserve, and that the mother is aware that relapses can occur at any time and are relatively common in the immediate postpartum period. In advanced cases the blood–brain barrier is functionally impaired, and care must be taken with local anaesthetic and opioid dosages.

Metabolic disease

Diabetes may be pre-existent, gestational, or the former revealed by the latter. Gestational diabetes is formally tested for after a failed glucose challenge (serum glucose >7.8 mmol/l 1 hour after 50 g oral glucose in a fasted patient). The formal test is a 100 g glucose load. The 'cut-offs' for a positive test are:

Fasting	5.8 mmol/l
1 hour	10.5 mmol/l
2 hours	9.2 mmol/l
3 hours	8.1 mmol/l

Diabetes mellitus is diagnosed if the 2-hour level is >11.1 mmol/l. Over 2 per cent of all pregnant women fall into the 8–11 mmol/l group, referred to as impaired glucose tolerance. Gestational diabetes carries increased risks for the mother and fetus unless control is good. This is usually achieved with dietary control alone, monitored with serial glucose, glycosylated haemoglobin (Hb A_{1C}) and weight recordings in a combined obstetric/endocrine clinic. Insulin therapy is started if normoglycaemia is not achieved. In labour, a sliding scale insulin infusion based on hourly blood glucose measurement combined with a 10 per cent dextrose and potassium infusion is required for insulin dependent gestational diabetics. Vaginal delivery may not be possible if the fetus is macrosomic. In mothers with longstanding diabetes the incidence of organ dysfunction is high, and should be documented and evaluated prenatally. Renal impairment is common, and hypertension and cardiac disease occur. Maternal diabetic nephropathy is associated with pre-eclampsia and with fetal complications, including prematurity (40–50 per cent), polyhydramnios (30 per cent), growth retardation (20 per cent) and fetal death (3 per cent).

- *Thyroid dysfunction* is uncommon during pregnancy. Hyperthyroidism is treated with carbimazole or propylthiouracil. Treatment is minimized to prevent fetal hypothyroidism, as both drugs cross the placenta. Symptoms improve through the second and third trimesters, and treatment can often be decreased or stopped. Partial thyroidectomy is occasionally required in the second trimester to control symptoms. *Hypothyroidism* is treated with thyroxine as normal, although closer monitoring is required to adjust doses.
- *Obesity* is a problem of the modern world and of pregnancy. The combination of these two leads to a proportion of morbidly obese patients presenting in labour or for Caesarean section. Regional anaesthesia offers obvious advantages in both cases, but is often technically extremely challenging. Risks of complications are increased, particularly deep venous thrombosis and pulmonary embolism, and wound dehiscence.

Haematological disease

The management of *sickle cell anaemia* in labour is similar in principle to that in the non-gravid population. Good hydration and oxygenation are essential to prevent sickling. Epidural analgesia is ideal to reduce stress, but the patient must be encouraged to keep mobile to decrease the risk of venous stasis and aortocaval compression. The management of a *sickle crisis* is an emergency section as soon as is practical, as placental blood flow can be seriously impaired.

Other congenital haematological disorders (*haemoglobinopathies, thalassaemias, factor deficiencies*) should be co-managed with haematologists throughout pregnancy. Epidural analgesia is usually no problem, but provision of fresh frozen plasma or factor concentrates may be necessary first.

Infective disease

Infectious diseases are neither more common nor more virulent in pregnancy. However, the presence of disease may have implications for the fetus and attending staff. *Universal precautions* (see Box 12.6) should always be taken, and should be part of routine practice for all staff. The Association of Anaesthetists of Great Britain and Ireland publishes guidelines on the subject.

- *Tuberculosis*, a disease thought to be dying out in the western world 15 years ago, is now increasingly common amongst first-generation immigrant parturients and the immunosuppressed. Provided active disease is not present, these patients present no risk to those around them. If doubt exists, full barrier precautions must be taken and an urgent referral to the local infectious disease team made.
- *HIV* infection is increasingly common in first-generation African immigrant communities and in intravenous drug users. Most obstetric units routinely test for HIV at booking, and zidovudine therapy is shown to decrease the incidence of vertical transmission from mother to fetus. Fetal monitoring cannot be invasive (scalp electrodes or scalp blood sampling) as this exposes the fetus to increased risk of infection. Elective Caesarean delivery reduces vertical transmission risk by over 20 per cent. Full barrier precautions should be taken in labour and at section, as a large amount of infected fluid is released. Epidural or subarachnoid anaesthesia is not contraindicated normally. In those with advanced, symptomatic disease, coagulopathy should be excluded. Any peripheral neuropathy should be documented prior to analgesic intervention. Cerebral toxoplasmosis can cause raised intracranial pressure, and in these cases regional analgesia is not appropriate.
- *Viral hepatitis* represents little medical challenge to the anaesthetist other than a need for scrupulous care when dealing with infected sharps. Severe clinical disease is rare in pregnancy, but serial liver function tests and clotting assays are of use in assessing disease progression.
- *Genital herpes simplex* infection, if active at the time of delivery, is an absolute indication for Caesarean section to prevent fetal infection.

Box 12.6. Universal precautions for blood-borne viral infections

- Use blunt needles/quills for drawing up drugs.
- Do not resheathe sharps.
- Dispose of sharps immediately after use in a proper, marked container.
- Pass sharps via a tray, not hand-to-hand.
- Always wear gloves for clinical procedures, and add a gown, mask and goggles if blood spillage is likely.
- Change gloves immediately if contaminated, and automatically before handling notes or between cases.
- Dress all skin abrasions with a waterproof dressing.
- Clean all blood spills properly in accordance with local policy.
- Label all laboratory specimens known to be infected as such.

'Anaesthetic' diseases

- Patients presenting antenatally or perinatally with a history of *suxamethonium apnoea, malignant hyperpyrexia* or *anaesthetic drug allergy* should be treated as usual – regional analgesia or anaesthesia is the ideal option for all interventions. The covering consultant should be informed that a patient with one of these conditions is on the labour ward. Care should be taken to use an uncontaminated oxygen supply in malignant hyperpyrexics (wall oxygen rather than the fresh gas outlet on the machine). If general anaesthesia is required in a patient with suxamethonium apnoea several options are available – to use the suxamethonium anyway for its speed of onset and be prepared to ventilate the mother electively postoperatively; to use a non-depolarizing relaxant with fast onset (such as rocuronium); or to use high-dose opioid (alfentanil or remifentanil) in place of a muscle relaxant.
- *Latex allergy* is an increasingly common problem. Latex-free equipment is available in the UK, and must be ordered in advance where the allergy is known.

Drug abuse

Chronic drug abusers represent a challenge in labour. Those using heroin or other opioids should be converted onto methadone, ideally preconception but usually in early pregnancy. In labour, analgesia can be a problem both in terms of pain control and intravenous access. It is indefensible to site an epidural for labour without large-bore intravenous access, whatever the mother has requested or says she will agree to!

Epidural analgesia is likely to be much more effective than intramuscular pethidine for labour pain. Methadone can be taken as usual. Ensure that the neonatal unit is fully aware, as the baby will have to be watched for evidence of withdrawal.

Cocaine and its derivatives and amphetamines may cause hypertension, tachyarrhythmia and confusion if taken during or just prior to labour. Marijuana is unlikely to cause significant problems.

13

Maternal and perinatal audit

Audit into morbidity and mortality should be a constant cycle that aims to improve the quality of care given to mothers. Most units collect outcome data relating to the numbers of general and regional anaesthetic procedures performed and complications that arise. Internal audit into complications should be continuous, and nationally there have been recommendations that the rate of post dural puncture headache should be less than 1 per cent of the epidurals performed. Ideally, of course, it should be zero. All other major complications, such as anaphylaxis, failed intubation, aspiration, haemorrhage and massive spinal anaesthesia, should be analysed in depth, and discussion as to whether equipment can be improved or whether the anaesthetist could have improved the care given to the patient should ensue. There are moves for a 'near miss' register to be instituted, because at present the national audits have maternal and infant mortality as the only final outcome measure.

Maternal mortality

Reports on Confidential Enquiries into Maternal Deaths have been produced triennially since 1952 in England and Wales (since 1956 for Northern Ireland and since 1965 for Scotland). A single 3-yearly report has been produced for the United Kingdom since 1985. Anonymous data are collected from obstetricians, general practitioners, midwives, health visitors, anaesthetists, pathologists, procurators fiscal and coroners, and a similarly composed group of local and central assessors review the information.

The aims and objectives of the Enquiries are five-fold:

1 To assess the causes and trends of maternal deaths whilst identifying avoidable or substandard factors
2 To reduce morbidity and mortality rates
3 To recommend improvements in clinical care and service provision
4 To suggest areas for future audit and research

5 To produce a triennial Report for the Chief Medical Officers of the United Kingdom.

Several definitions are elucidated in Box 13.1. Maternal deaths are divided into direct, indirect, late, and fortuitous deaths.

The number of deaths has decreased since 1952 to the present level of about 10–12 deaths per 100 000 maternities (defined as the number of pregnancies resulting in live births or stillbirths after or at 24 weeks' gestation). The leading causes of death (Box 13.2) are thromboembolism, hypertensive disorders, amniotic fluid embolism, early pregnancy (ectopic, abortion), sepsis, haemorrhage and anaesthesia. Death rates are higher in primiparous women over 35 years of age. Black patients have a three-fold greater risk of maternal mortality.

The reports give guidance on the management of conditions, but still about 40 per cent of deaths are due to substandard care. The main causes of substandard care are:

- The failure of junior staff to diagnose problems early and refer to senior doctors
- The failure of consultants to attend, and inappropriate delegation of responsibility
- A lack of clear guidelines or policies on the management of

---

Box 13.1. Definitions of maternal deaths

- Maternal death: the death of a woman while pregnant or within 42 days of termination of pregnancy, from any cause related to or aggravated by the pregnancy or its management, but not from accidental or incidental causes.
- Direct death: death resulting from obstetric complications of the pregnant state, from interventions, omissions, incorrect treatment, or a chain of events resulting from any of the above.
- Indirect death: death arising from previous existing disease, or disease that developed in pregnancy and was not due to direct obstetric causes but which was aggravated by the physiological effects of pregnancy.
- Late death: death occurring between 42 days and 1 year from the termination of pregnancy that is due to direct or indirect maternal causes.
- Fortuitous death: death from unrelated causes that happen to occur in pregnancy or the puerperium.

Box 13.2. Main direct maternal deaths: causes from four triennial reports (1973–1975 for England and Wales, the remainder for the United Kingdom)

Causes	1973–75	1988–90	1991–93	1993–96
Hypertensive disease	34 (15%)	27 (19%)	20 (16%)	20 (15%)
Thromboembolism	34 (15%)	33 (23%)	35 (27%)	48 (36%)
Haemorrhage	21 (9%)	22 (15%)	15 (12%)	12 (9%)
Early pregnancy (ectopic)	19 (8%)	15 (10%)	9 (7%)	12 (9%)
Amniotic fluid embolism	14 (6%)	11 (8%)	10 (8%)	17 (13%)
Sepsis	19 (8%)	7 (5%)	9 (7%)	14 (11%)
Anaesthesia	27 (12%)	4 (3%)	8 (6%)	1 (<1%)
Total	227	145	129	134

conditions such as haemorrhage, pulmonary embolism and eclampsia
- A failure of team work
- Failure of the lead clinician to identify and appropriately refer rare conditions and diseases.

Recent recommendations include the wider use of thrombophylaxis, and better investigation and diagnosis of patients with suspected embolism. Other important general recommendations include the ongoing use and proven benefit of prophylactic antibiotics in Caesarean section, the seeking of early microbial advice, and the use of parenteral antibiotics before diagnosis confirmation in sepsis. Haemolytic streptococcal infection is still common.

The deaths from anaesthesia appear to be decreasing, but there is no room for complacency. Historically, anaesthesia was always the third most common cause of maternal death, but it is now at the lower end on the scale of causes of maternal mortality. Most deaths have occurred as a result of the complications of general anaesthesia (failure to intubate, hypoxia and aspiration), but deaths are also reported from the complications of regional anaesthesia. Recent recommendations to improve care include adequate consultant involvement, adequate recovery, high dependency and the availability of intensive care facilities, the use of appropriate monitoring equipment (capnography, oximetry), appropriate antacid therapy, appropriate anaesthetic assistance, and the education of midwives in recovery and high dependency care.

Perinatal mortality

The Confidential Enquiries into Stillbirths and Deaths in Infancy was established in 1992 to improve understanding of how the risks of death in late fetal life up to infancy might be reduced. The aim is to identify and highlight risks that can be attributed to suboptimal clinical care. The causes of perinatal mortality are mainly hypoxia, low birth weight and congenital abnormalities. Again, these yearly reports emphasize that deaths result from a failure of communication, a lack of training, and an absence of clear clinical guidelines. The 7th Annual Report focused on anaesthesia, and 25 anaesthetic incidents were reviewed. Deaths arose from the serious complications related to general anaesthesia, delays with personnel, and the delays in the provision of either general or regional anaesthesia once the anaesthetist was available. The largest contributing factor to deaths in babies is delay in 'team' assembly. Ideally a resident dedicated anaesthetist of more than 1 year's training and a dedicated anaesthetic assistant should be provided for all consultant-led units. The degree of urgency of the need to deliver the baby is not always made clear to the anaesthetist, and occasionally an inappropriate choice of anaesthetic technique can be made. Delay in delivery was attributed to the management of anaphylaxis in the mother in two cases. Rapid delivery of the fetus should not be delayed whilst 'stabilization' of the mother occurs. A rapid delivery has no deleterious effect on the resuscitation of the mother and may even aid maternal resuscitation. In severe anaphylaxis, epinephrine is the drug treatment of choice and may improve rather than reduce uteroplacental blood flow. It is recommended that audit of the time it takes to set up successful anaesthesia for emergency Caesarean section should take place. This is defined as less than 30 minutes, but this time is considered 'pragmatic' rather than evidence-based, and obviously depends upon how urgent the Caesarean section is.

14

Maternal and neonatal resuscitation

Anaesthetists in maternity units work with staff unfamiliar with the management of maternal cardiac arrest. Despite regular staff training sessions, the anaesthetist is the pivotal member of the maternal resuscitation team and should take the lead. A dedicated paediatric registrar and senior house officer usually staff neonatal units in large centres. However, the attending paediatrician at deliveries is often the most junior, and thus it may fall to the anaesthetist to assist in the early stages of neonatal resuscitation.

Maternal cardiac arrest

The cause of a cardiac arrest must be determined and all possible causes treated (see Box 14.1). There are two important features of maternal resuscitation that need to be carried out in addition to both basic and advanced life support. First, cardiopulmonary resuscitation (CPR) will be unsuccessful if venous return is impaired, and this occurs if the pregnant patient is resuscitated in the supine position. It is imperative that the cardiac arrest be managed with the patient in a partial left lateral position or, using a

---

Box 14.1. Causes of maternal cardiac arrest

- Airway – oedema, obstruction, misplaced or dislodged tube at general anaesthetic Caesarean section.
- Breathing – bronchospasm, pneumothorax.
- Circulatory – cardiovascular collapse: cardiogenic (dysrhythmia, exacerbation of pre-existing condition, infarction, valvular disease); septic (chorioamnionitis, sepsis not related to pregnancy); hypovolaemic (haemorrhage, concealed/revealed, antepartum/postpartum).
- Embolism – clot (from deep vein thrombosis), amniotic fluid.
- Anaesthesia – *epidural*, total spinal, intravenous injection; *general anaesthesia*, intubation problems, anaphylaxis, equipment/monitoring failure, malignant hyperpyrexia.
- Drugs – anaphylaxis.
- Cerebral – bleeding, infection, infarction, seizure.

'human wedge', with the patient positioned in a left lateral tilt. This can be achieved by having an assistant kneel with his or her buttocks resting on the heels; the patient can then be propped over the thighs of the assistant and thus maintained in a stable, tilted position for CPR. Secondly, the baby needs to be delivered by Caesarean section immediately. A well-managed maternal cardiac arrest should lead to the delivery of a live infant and improves the prospect of successful maternal outcome.

Maternal anaphylaxis

This is no more or less rare an event in pregnancy or labour than in non-gravid patients. The main signs are bronchospasm, flushing, hypotension and tachycardia, and fetal distress will onset rapidly in the presence of hypoxia and reduced placental blood flow. Treatment is summarized in Box 14.2, and follow-up in Box 14.3.

Neonatal resuscitation

Most newborn babies establish respiration spontaneously after delivery, and the only care required initially is to dry and wrap the infant. Although deliveries in which a greater degree of support than this is required can be anticipated (see Box 14.4), fetal problems are often sudden and unexpected, so all should be familiar with the resuscitation equipment and protocol. It is vital to remember that the anaesthetist has a primary ethical and legal concern for the mother. If assisting in the neonatal resuscitation potentially jeopardizes the mother (e.g. active bleeding), the anaesthetist must not get involved with the care of a second patient.

Apgar scoring (see Box 14.5) is the most commonly used system for neonatal assessment. It is quick, and provides a clear guide to the status of the fetus. It is routinely recorded at 1 and 5 minutes post-delivery. Any child who has a reduced Apgar score at delivery (i.e. less than 10/10) should be urgently assessed and treated appropriately.

Airway

The optimum position of the neonatal airway differs from the 'sniffing the morning air' position in the adult because of the large size of the head in general, and the occiput in particular, compared to the body. The infant should be flat on his or her back with the neck extended. Modern paediatric resuscitaires have a sloped leading edge to facilitate this position. If breathing

---

Box 14.2. Anaphylaxis in pregnancy: treatment

Immediate:
- Stop suspected cause (drugs, latex).
- Call for help.
- Start CPR if necessary; position mother in lateral tilt, elevate legs.
- Ensure good airway, 100 per cent oxygen, large-bore intravenous access, monitoring.
- Epinephrine 50–100 μg (0.5–1 ml 1 : 10 000 solution) bolus doses as required, and start fast intravenous crystalloid infusion.
- Consider emergency Caesarean section.

Continuing treatment:
- Further epinephrine bolus doses if required.
- Consider: salbutamol nebulizer 5 mg for bronchospasm; antihistamine (chlorpheniramine 10 mg intravenously); steroids (hydrocortisone 200 mg intravenously).
- Blood tests: arterial gases, urea and electrolytes, full blood count, clotting and serum to save for later investigation (serum tryptase, immunoglobulin levels).
- ITU/HDU admission.

Box 14.3. Anaphylaxis in pregnancy: follow-up

- Allergy skin testing.
- Immunological consultation re: assays for Ig E, IgM.
- Full discussion and documentation of results; copies to patient, GP and hospital notes.
- Medical alert bracelet for patient.

---

does not commence immediately, gently reposition the child and suck out any mucus, fluid or meconium present in the mouth, nose or pharynx.

Breathing

The first breath a baby takes is the most difficult, as this expands the collapsed lungs by overcoming the high surface fluid tension within. This forces any remaining alveolar fluid into the circulation and drops the high pulmonary artery pressure, leading to establishment of normal cardiopulmonary circulatory flow. If respiratory effort is poor or the infant is centrally cyanosed, continuous positive airway

---

Box 14.4. Prenatal predictors of a need for fetal resuscitation

- Fetal distress.
- Meconium-stained amniotic fluid (particularly if thick and fresh).
- Abnormal antenatal scans.
- Abnormal presentation.
- Multiple delivery.
- Premature delivery.

Box 14.5. Neonatal Apgar scores

	Score		
Clinical sign	0	1	2
Heart rate (beats/min)	No pulse	<100	>100
Respiratory eort	Apnoea	Poor	Good
Colour (mucous membranes)	White	Blue	Pink
Muscle tone	Flaccid	Poor	Normal
Response to stimulation	None	Grimace	Cry

---

pressure (CPAP) is helpful both to improve oxygenation and to help expand the collapsed alveoli in the lungs. If the child fails to rapidly improve, is apnoeic or has a heart rate of less than 100 beats/min, formal ventilation should be started and the neonatal crash team alerted. Once the baby is oxygenated, intubation with an uncuffed endotracheal tube should be performed (size 3.5 mm ID in a term infant, 3.0 mm ID if small-for-dates or premature, and the tube should be no further than 4 cm at the cords to prevent accidental endobronchial intubation). A straight-bladed laryngoscope is all that is available usually – this is used to directly lift the epiglottis. Ventilatory rates of 30–40 breaths per minute are used for facemask or endotracheal ventilation.

Circulation
The neonatal heart rate is best assessed with a stethoscope or by palpating the umbilical cord at its base. If the heart rate is less than 60 beats/min, or less than 100 with poor respiratory effort or cyanosis, external cardiac massage must be commenced and the neonatal crash team alerted. Massage should be performed with

the thumbs over the lower half of the sternum and the hands round the chest. The chest should be compressed by 2–3 cm, 120–140 times per minute.

Unless there is an underlying cardiac or metabolic abnormality, virtually all neonatal arrests are secondary to hypoxia. Resumption of respiration and the restoration of a good cardiac output usually follow rapidly once adequate oxygenation is ensured.

Intravenous access

In the resuscitation context, the umbilical vein is by far the easiest route of access to the neonatal circulation. It can easily be identified in the cord as a large blue superficial structure. If the cord is held taut between the operator's forefinger and thumb, an incision can be made in the cord and an umbilical vein catheter passed. A ligature is then applied proximal to the incision. Blood should be taken for blood count, electrolytes, cross-match and sugar. Neonates are prone to hypoglycaemia and this needs careful observation, especially in macrosomic babies. Common resuscitation drugs and their dosages are included in Box 14.6.

Meconium

If meconium-stained liquor is seen during labour, an experienced resuscitator should be present at delivery. The mouth, nose and pharynx of the child should be suctioned prior to the child taking its first breath whenever possible (after delivery of the head but before delivery of the body) to minimize the risk of aspiration. Suction on the resuscitaire runs at a smaller partial vacuum than normal suction, so care is needed if using normal suction not to occlude the pipe for long periods. If this procedure is successful and the baby is healthy, pink and vigorous, no further action is necessary. If aspiration is suspected, the infant should be intubated and the trachea suctioned directly using the endotracheal tube as a large suction catheter. Respiratory observation in the baby unit is vital after this, and prolonged ventilation is sometimes required.

Box 14.6. Neonatal resuscitation

- Intravenous fluid: give if capillary refill is prolonged or if fetal sepsis or hypovolaemia is suspected – colloid or blood 10 ml/kg (maximum two doses of colloid before considering blood, as there is the risk of dilutional anaemia).
- Epinephrine: 10 µg/kg endotracheally or intravenously, increase to 100 µg/kg on third dose (intravenous only). Note: 10 µg/kg = 0.1 ml of 1 : 10 000/kg (standard Minijet strength); 100 µg/kg = 1 ml of 1 : 10 000/kg (standard Minijet strength).
- Naloxone: 100 µg/kg intramuscularly. Any child given naloxone for opioid-induced respiratory depression must be admitted to a high dependency observation area, as the half-life of naloxone is much shorter than the half-life of most opioids administered in labour and further respiratory depression may occur.
- Defibrillation: 2 j/kg for the first two shocks, then 4 j/kg.
- Ventilation: rescuscitaires usually have two sources of ventilatory oxygen; a neonatal ambubag with a round facemask, and a pipeline connector with a variable blow-off valve – after connection to the tube occlusion applies a pressure to the valve limit. The valve is usually left at 15–20 cmH$_2$O.
- Heat: neonates cool rapidly due to evaporative heat loss if damp, their high surface-to-volume ratio, and impaired metabolic compensation. They should be vigorously dried as soon as possible after delivery, then wrapped in warm, dry blankets. The radiant heater on the resuscitaire is designed to keep the baby at a skin temperature of 33–35°C.

15

Anaesthesia for surgery during pregnancy

Surgery is increasingly common during pregnancy, both for problems relating to the pregnancy and for emergency treatment of conditions not associated with the pregnancy. The overall quoted incidence of antenatal surgery is of the order of 1 per cent. As a rule, anaesthesia should be regional wherever possible and should be avoided completely (barring emergencies) in the first 8–10 weeks, during organogenesis.

Antenatal surgery related to the pregnancy

- Undoubtedly the commonest operative procedure carried out is *termination of pregnancy*. The legal gestational limit on this operation currently stands at 24 weeks' gestation, but in practice most terminations are within the first trimester. The anaesthetic and surgical requirements for this are the same as for *evacuation of retained products of conception* (ERPC) after an incomplete abortion. The patient should be fasted for at least 6 hours. Regional anaesthesia is adequate with a block to at least T_8, but general anaesthesia is more commonly used for psychological reasons. Ventilation is usually unnecessary, anaesthesia being maintained using a volatile agent or propofol infusion/bolus technique on a laryngeal mask or facemask with the patient breathing spontaneously. The use of total intravenous anaesthesia is advantageous in that it avoids the uterine relaxant effects of volatile anaesthetic agents, thus decreasing the risk of bleeding after curettage. In the absence of symptoms requiring intubation (reflux, emergency procedure etc.) it is widely held that patients at 15 weeks' or less gestation are at no increased risk of aspiration, and some authorities would argue 20 weeks' gestation as a safe limit. For those at risk, antacid prophylaxis (ranitidine 150 mg and metoclopramide 10 mg orally at least 1 hour preoperatively, and sodium citrate 0.3 M 30 ml immediately prior to induction) and rapid sequence induction after pre-oxygenation should be used.

- Some patients with cervical incompetence require insertion of a *Shirodkar suture*. This is a ribbon-like suture tied through the cervix at operation, and is said to increase the fetal survival through prevention of premature delivery from 20 per cent to 80 per cent. Spinal anaesthesia is ideal for this procedure.

- *Reversal of female circumcision* is an increasingly common operation in areas with a high immigrant population from sub-Saharan Africa. The circumcision is performed in childhood, and varies in severity from a simple suturing together of part of the labia majora to complete excision of all external genitalia (akin to a radical vulvectomy). Reversal can be performed under regional anaesthesia, where 1–1.5 ml heavy bupivacaine 0.5% will provide a good 'saddle' block, but postoperative pain can be severe. In some centres the reversal is carried out during labour, but this is suboptimal, as vaginal examination is impossible in these cases prior to reversal.

- Surgery for *ectopic pregnancy* ranges in severity and urgency from an abnormal ultrasound finding in an asymptomatic patient to an emergency, life-saving procedure when the ectopic ruptures, causing torrential haemorrhage. Deaths from this condition have fallen over the last 10 years, and currently run at three to four per 1000 cases in the UK. Deaths are almost universally related to substandard care, particularly relating to lack of speed in diagnosis leading to death from haemorrhage and its complications. In asymptomatic patients, surgery is semi-elective and aimed at conservation of the fallopian tube. In emergency cases, aggressive fluid resuscitation and invasive monitoring are vital, and senior gynaecological and anaesthetic support should be sought early. In these cases laparoscopic surgery is not appropriate, as it will be technically difficult and slower, and the gas insufflation required may further reduce venous return, leading to cardiovascular collapse.

Surgery not related to pregnancy

Elective surgery is almost never performed during pregnancy because of the increased risk of spontaneous abortion. The cause of this is unclear but is thought to be related to a variety of factors, including the stress response to surgery, pressor responses during anaesthesia and surgery, and the systemic effects of general

---

Box 15.1. Principles of surgery in the gravid patient

- Avoid surgery if possible, particularly in the first 8–10 weeks.
- Avoid general anaesthesia if possible.
- Consider drug eects on the fetus and placenta (avoid drugs aecting placental perfusion, check all drugs for potential fetal eects etc.).
- Use a lateral wedge or tilt if over 20 weeks' gestation to prevent aortocaval compression.
- Consider tocolytic therapy if abdominal surgery, and steroid therapy to mature fetal lung tissue.
- Ensure adequate fetal monitoring.

---

anaesthesia. First trimester anaesthesia is particularly to be avoided, as there is some suggestion of increased teratogenic risk, shown in rats with nitrous oxide.

If the pregnancy is non-viable, concern should be focused solely on the mother. If a normal pregnancy is ongoing, surgery should be delayed where possible until fetal viability is improved (> 32 weeks' gestation) and steroids should be given preoperatively according to local guidelines to improve fetal lung maturity. The neonatal unit should be forewarned. The principles of surgery in the gravid patient are summarized in Box 15.1.

Fetal surgery

This is a new field with huge potential for development. In utero surgery is improving technically with advances in laparoscopic techniques. The prevention of fetal movement and distress is achieved via transplacental drug effects, but increasing efforts are being made to use direct fetal drug administration.

Further reading

Bonica, J. J. and McDonald, J. S. (eds) (1995) Principles and Practice of Obstetric Analgesia and Anesthesia, 2nd edn. Williams and Wilkins.

Gambling, D. R. and Douglas, M. J. (eds) (1998) Obstetric Anesthesia and Uncommon Disorders. WB Saunders Co.

Russell, I. F. and Lyons, G. (eds) (1997) Clinical Problems in Obstetric Anaesthesia. Chapman Hall Medical.

Van Zunden, A. and Ostheimer, G. W. (eds) (1996) Pain Relief and Anaesthesia in Obstetrics. Churchill Livingstone.

Index

Printed in the United Kingdom
by Lightning Source UK Ltd.
124299UK00001B/31/A